THE EVERYTHING GUIDE TO THE KETOGENIC DIET

Dear Reader,

When I started college, I was fully on board the low-fat diet train. I wanted to make sure that I stayed healthy and avoided that dreaded "freshman 15," and limiting fat was the only way to do that, right? I stocked my fridge with low-fat flavored yogurts and low-fat nutrition bars. I got low-fat peanut butter and swapped out my butter for a miraculous butter-like substance that contained no calories and, you guessed it, no fat!

Fast forward to one year later and not only did I gain the freshman 15 and then some, but I was left feeling sluggish, tired, bloated, and constipated. I could barely wake up for my classes in the morning, and when I was able to drag myself to class, my energy was so low and my concentration was so lacking that I couldn't even pay attention. I knew something needed to change.

I started doing my own nutrition research—this was actually what started me on my path to becoming a nutrition consultant—and couldn't believe all the misinformation that I had been fed. I found out that not only is fat vital to optimal body functioning, it can actually help promote weight loss. I switched my focus from low-fat foods to taking in plenty of healthy fats and limiting carbohydrates—the basics of a ketogenic diet—and began to feel so much better. My energy levels stabilized, the excess weight came off, and I was able to concentrate—and excel—in class once again.

Whether you're new to the ketogenic diet or just refreshing your memory, one of the most important things to take away from this book is that fat is not the enemy. In fact, it should be one of your most important allies.

I wish you all the best in health and in life.

Lindsay Boyers, CHNC

Welcome to the EVERYTHING® Series!

These handy, accessible books give you all you need to tackle a difficult project, gain a new hobby, comprehend a fascinating topic, prepare for an exam, or even brush up on something you learned back in school but have since forgotten.

You can choose to read an Everything® book from cover to cover or just pick out the information you want from our four useful boxes: e-questions, e-facts, e-alerts, and e-ssentials.

We give you everything you need to know on the subject, but throw in a lot of fun stuff along the way, too.

We now have more than 400 Everything® books in print, spanning such wide-ranging categories as weddings, pregnancy, cooking, music instruction, foreign language, crafts, pets, New Age, and so much more. When you're done reading them all, you can finally say you know Everything®!

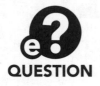

QUESTION

Answers to
common questions

FACT

Important snippets
of information

ALERT

Urgent
warnings

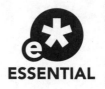

ESSENTIAL

Quick
handy tips

PUBLISHER Karen Cooper

MANAGING EDITOR, EVERYTHING® SERIES Lisa Laing

COPY CHIEF Casey Ebert

ASSISTANT PRODUCTION EDITOR Alex Guarco

ACQUISITIONS EDITOR Hillary Thompson

DEVELOPMENT EDITOR Eileen Mullan

EVERYTHING® SERIES COVER DESIGNER Erin Alexander

Visit the entire Everything® series at *www.everything.com*

THE
EVERYTHING®
GUIDE TO THE
KETOGENIC DIET

A step-by-step guide to the ultimate
fat-burning diet plan!

Lindsay Boyers, CHNC

Adams Media
New York London Toronto Sydney New Delhi

To Gianna and Gabriella. I love you.

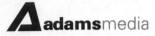

Adams Media
An Imprint of Simon & Schuster, Inc.
57 Littlefield Street
Avon, Massachusetts 02322

An Everything® Series Book.
Everything® and everything.com® are registered trademarks of Simon & Schuster, Inc.

ADAMS MEDIA and colophon are trademarks of Simon and Schuster.

For information about special discounts for bulk purchases, please contact Simon & Schuster Special Sales at 1-866-506-1949 or business@simonandschuster.com.

The Simon & Schuster Speakers Bureau can bring authors to your live event. For more information or to book an event contact the Simon & Schuster Speakers Bureau at 1-866-248-3049 or visit our website at www.simonspeakers.com.

Manufactured in the United States of America

10

Library of Congress Cataloging-in-Publication Data has been applied for.

ISBN 978-1-4405-8691-0
ISBN 978-1-4405-8692-7 (ebook)

Contains material adapted and abridged from *The Everything® Slow Cooker Cookbook* by Margaret Kaeter, copyright © 2002 by Simon & Schuster, Inc., ISBN 13: 978-1-58062-667-5; *The Everything® Slow Cooking for a Crowd Cookbook* by Katie Thompson, copyright © 2005 by Simon & Schuster, Inc., ISBN 13: 978-1-59337-391-7; *The Everything® Green Smoothies Book* by Britt Brandon with Lorena Novak Bull, copyright © 2011 by Simon & Schuster, Inc., ISBN 13: 978-1-4405-2564-3; *The Everything® Indian Slow Cooker Cookbook* by Prerna Singh, copyright © 2012 by Simon & Schuster, Inc., ISBN 13: 978-1-4405-4168-1; *The Everything® Nordic Cookbook* by Kari Schoening Diehl, copyright © 2012 by Simon & Schuster, Inc., ISBN 13: 978-1-4405-3186-6; and *The Everything® Brazilian Cookbook* by Marian Blazes, copyright © 2014 by Simon & Schuster, Inc., ISBN 13: 978-1-4405-7938-7.

Contents

Acknowledgments

Thank you to my family—my mom, Lola; my dad, Scott; my sister, Tiffany; and my brother, Sean—for your unwavering support as I worked on this book—and always. Thank you to Paul for always being there for me when I need you. I love you all. Thank you to Hillary Thompson for giving me this opportunity and for helping me to see it through from start to finish. Thank you to Eileen Mullan for your editing expertise.

Introduction

IN THE 1990S, FAT was demonized. The macronutrient became the dirty word of the nutrition industry, and was shunned by consumers and professionals alike. Many believed that fat was the primary cause of a host of health problems, including weight gain, high cholesterol, and heart disease, although there wasn't—and still isn't—any sufficient scientific evidence to support these claims. Despite what the science showed, however, people began jumping on the low-fat bandwagon, turning to low-fat alternatives that were loaded with sugar and carbohydrates instead. As more fat-free and low-fat products became available, the average American became bigger. By 2001, about one-third of the American population was overweight. The prevalence of heart disease increased and diabetes rates soared. So what went wrong?

Fresh whole foods such as meat, eggs, cream, and butter—the foods your ancestors ate for centuries—were being replaced with low-fat Frankenfoods such as margarine, low-fat snack cookies, and skim milk. These foods were not only full of sugar and carbohydrates; some were also loaded with artificial ingredients. When these substances are consumed regularly, over time, the human body reacts by gaining weight, showing symptoms of fatigue and brain fog, and succumbing to chronic conditions. Although scientific research produced findings to the contrary, fat—especially saturated fat—had developed a lasting reputation for being bad for you. Although the low-fat diet craze eventually dwindled, the damage was done. Fat was shunned.

Now this may shock you—after all, it's likely that you've been told for years or even decades to eat plenty of whole-grain carbohydrates and avoid saturated fat like the plague—but fat is good for you. Fat, even, perhaps especially, saturated fat, helps your body run like a well-oiled machine. Your body's need for fat is the basis of the ketogenic diet, which encourages that you get most of your calories—around 75 percent—from fat and only 5 to 10 percent from carbohydrates. The remaining calories come from high-quality proteins.

The ketogenic diet is not a new trend or a fad diet. It's actually been around for decades. It was used in the 1920s as the main treatment method for difficult-to-control epilepsy in young children—and it worked remarkably well. Eventually, it fell out of fashion with the increasing availability of anti-seizure medications. People preferred a quick fix even if that fix meant the potential for more side effects. Today, people following nutritional ketogenic diets report weight loss, increased energy levels, better mood, improved concentration, and mental clarity.

Nevertheless, mainstream media and even some healthcare professionals tend to present the ketogenic diet in a negative light. Like fat, ketones, which are compounds created when the body begins using fat instead of carbohydrates for energy, have a bad reputation. Most of the concerns surrounding ketones and the ketogenic diet are unfounded or are a result of confusion between the terms "ketosis" and "ketoacidosis." The *European Journal of Clinical Nutrition* states that this confusion and preconceived notions about the ketogenic diet—like the idea that all fat is bad for you— may be "presenting unnecessary barriers to their use as therapeutic tools in the physician's hand."

So now let's put the rumors to rest and understand why fat is not just good but is essential to maintaining optimal health. It's actually sugar, carbohydrates, and processed vegetable oils that are largely responsible for weight gain and the increasing rates of chronic health conditions. Limiting carbohydrates and replacing them with both saturated and unsaturated fats—the basis of the ketogenic diet—can not only help you lose weight, it can help you stay healthy for years to come.

CHAPTER 1

Understanding Ketosis

Your body is highly intelligent. It knows exactly what it wants and what it needs to do to get what it wants, and the main thing it wants is energy. Without energy, your cells would starve and you would die. In order to make sure that it always has access to energy, your body has several metabolic pathways it can use to convert the food you eat into useable energy. The default metabolic pathway is one that uses the glucose from carbohydrates as fuel. As long as you provide your body with carbohydrates, it will use them as energy, storing fat in the process. When you deny your body carbohydrates, it has to turn somewhere else to get the energy it needs to live.

What Is Ketosis?

Your body's second preferred source of energy is fat; when carbohydrates are not easily accessible, your body turns to fat to get the energy it needs. When this happens, the liver breaks down fat into fatty acids and then breaks down these fatty acids into an energy-rich substance called ketones or ketone bodies. The presence of ketone bodies in the blood is called ketosis. The goal of a ketogenic diet is to kick your body into long-term ketosis, essentially turning it into a fat-burning machine.

How Your Body Obtains Energy

Your cells need a constant supply of energy to stay alive and keep you alive. Even when you're sitting on the couch doing nothing, your body is generating energy for your cells. Since energy cannot be created, only converted from one form to another, your body needs to get this energy from somewhere, so it uses the food you eat. Your body can use each macronutrient—carbohydrates, fat, and protein—for energy. The biochemical process of obtaining energy is a complicated one, but it's important to understand the basics so you can get a feel for how ketosis works on a cellular level.

Energy from Protein

Protein is the body's least favorite macronutrient to use as energy. This is because protein serves so many other functions in the body, way more than any other macronutrient. Protein provides structural support to every cell in your body and helps maintain your body tissues. Proteins act as enzymes that play a role in all of the chemical reactions in your body. Without these enzymes, these chemical reactions would be so slow that your body wouldn't be able to carry out basic processes like digestion and metabolism and you wouldn't be able to survive. Proteins also help maintain fluid and acid-base balance, help transport substances such as oxygen through the body and waste out of the body, and act as antibodies to keep your immune system strong and help fight off illness.

ESSENTIAL

This process of using protein for energy is what makes extreme calorie restriction dangerous. When your diet doesn't provide enough calories, your body begins to break down the protein in your muscles for energy, which can lead to muscle loss or muscle wasting in addition to nutritional deficiencies.

Proteins are made up of amino acids. When you eat proteins, your body breaks them down into their individual amino acids, which are then converted into sugars through a process called deamination. Your body can use these protein-turned-sugars as a form of energy, but that means your body isn't using the amino acids for those other important functions. It's best to avoid forcing the body to use protein for energy, and you do that by providing it with the other nutrients it needs. That being said, if the body has no other choice but to use protein for energy, it will.

Energy from Carbohydrates

Although your body is adept at using any food that's available for energy, it always turns to carbohydrates first. When you eat carbohydrates, they are broken down into glucose or another sugar that's easily converted to glucose. Glucose is absorbed through the walls of the small intestine and then enters your body by way of your bloodstream, which causes your blood glucose levels to rise. As soon as the glucose enters your blood, your pancreas sends out insulin to pick up the sugar and carry it to your cells so they can use it as energy.

Once your cells have used all the glucose they need at that time, much of the remaining glucose is converted into glycogen (the storage form of glucose), which is then stored in the liver and muscles. The liver has a limited ability to store glycogen, though; it can only store enough glycogen to provide you with energy for about 24 hours. All the extra glucose that can't be stored is converted into triglycerides, the storage form of fat, and stored in your fat cells.

A healthy adult can store about 500 grams (2,000 calories worth) of carbohydrates. Approximately 400 grams are stored as glycogen in your muscles; 90–110 grams are stored as glycogen in the liver; and 25 grams circulate throughout the bloodstream as glucose. Your body has an unlimited ability to store fat.

When you don't eat for a few hours and your blood sugar starts to drop, your body will call on the glycogen stored in the liver and muscles for energy before anything else. The pancreas releases a hormone called glucagon, which triggers the release of glucose from the glycogen stored in your liver to help raise your blood sugar levels. This process is called glycogenolysis. The glycogen stored in your liver is used exclusively to increase your blood glucose levels, while the glycogen stored in your muscles is used strictly as fuel for your muscles. When you eat carbohydrates again, your body uses the glucose it gets from them to replenish those glycogen stores. If you regularly eat carbohydrates, your body never has a problem getting access to glucose for energy and the stored fat stays where it is—in your fat cells.

Endurance athletes use the terms "hitting a wall" or "bonking" to describe the point at which they've depleted their glycogen stores and no longer have access to a quick form of energy. Bonking usually manifests as sudden fatigue or a complete loss of energy. When you see marathon runners drinking glucose shots during a race, it's because they want to replenish glycogen stores quickly so that they have enough energy to finish.

Energy from Fat

The body prefers to use carbohydrates for energy because they're easily accessible and fast-acting, but in the absence of carbohydrates, your body turns to fat. The fat from the food you eat is broken down into fatty acids, which enter the bloodstream through the walls of the small intestine. Most of your cells can directly use fatty acids for energy, but some specialized cells, such as the cells in your brain and your muscles, can't run on fatty acids directly. To appease these cells and give them the energy they need, your body uses fatty acids to make ketones.

The Creation of Ketones

When your body doesn't have access to glucose—for example, during times of fasting or when intentionally following a low-carbohydrate diet—it turns to fat for energy. Fat is taken to the liver where it is broken down into glycerol and fatty acids through a process called beta-oxidation. The fatty acid molecules are further broken down through a process called ketogenesis, and a specific ketone body called acetoacetate is formed.

Over time, as your body becomes adapted to using ketones as fuel, your muscles convert acetoacetate into beta-hydroxybutyrate or BHB, which is the preferred ketogenic source of energy for your brain, and acetone, most of which is expelled from the body as waste.

The glycerol created during beta-oxidation goes through a process called gluconeogenesis. During gluconeogenesis, the body converts glycerol into glucose that your body can use for energy. Your body can also convert excess protein into glucose. Your body does need some glucose to function, but it doesn't need carbohydrates to get it. It does a good job of converting whatever it can into the simple sugar.

Ketosis and Weight Loss

Now that you understand how your body creates energy and how ketones are formed, you may be left wondering how this translates into weight loss. When you eat a lot of carbohydrates, your body happily burns them for energy and stores any excess as glycogen in your liver or as triglycerides in your fat cells. When you take carbohydrates out of the equation, your body depletes its glycogen stores in the liver and muscles and then turns to fat for energy. Your body obtains energy from the fat in the food you eat, but it also uses the triglycerides, or fats, stored in your fat cells. When your body starts burning stored fat, your fat cells shrink and you begin to lose weight and become leaner.

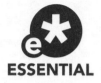

How to Induce Ketosis

Inducing ketosis is not an easy task, but once you get the hang of it, it can become second nature. The first step in inducing ketosis is to severely limit carbohydrate consumption, but that's not enough. You must limit your protein consumption as well. Traditional low-carbohydrate diets don't induce ketosis because they allow a high intake of protein. Because your body is able to convert excess protein into glucose, your body never switches over to burning fat as fuel. You can induce ketosis by following a high-fat diet that allows moderate amounts of protein and allows only a small amount of carbohydrates—or what is called a ketogenic diet.

The exact percentage of each macronutrient you need to kick your body into ketosis may vary from person to person, but in general, the macronutrient ratio falls into the following ranges:

- 60–75 percent of calories from fat
- 15–30 percent of calories from protein
- 5–10 percent of calories from carbohydrates

This largely differs from both a standard low-carbohydrate diet, which typically allows more calories to come from protein, and the traditional dietary reference intakes set by the Institute of Medicine.

Currently, the Institute of Medicine recommends getting 45–65 percent of your calories from carbohydrates, 20–35 percent of your calories from fat, and 10–35 percent of your calories from protein. Although the individual recommendations of low-carbohydrate diets differ based on which one you follow, they typically allow about 20 percent of calories from carbohydrates, 25–30 percent from protein, and 55–65 percent from fat.

Once you're in ketosis, you have to continue with the high-fat, low-carbohydrate, moderate-protein plan. Eating too many carbohydrates or too much protein can kick you out of ketosis at any time by providing your body with enough glucose to stop using fat as fuel.

Signs That You Are in Ketosis

Signs that you're in ketosis may start appearing after only one week of following a true ketogenic diet. For some people, it can take longer—as much as three months. The amount of time it takes for you to start seeing signs that your body is burning fat for fuel largely depends on you as an individual. When signs do start to show, they are pretty similar across the board.

Keto "Flu"

"Keto flu" or "low-carb flu" commonly affects people in the first few days of starting a ketogenic diet. Of course, the ketogenic diet doesn't actually cause the flu, but the phenomenon is given the term because its symptoms closely resemble that of the flu. It would be more accurate to refer to this stage as a carbohydrate withdrawal, because that's really what it is. When you take carbohydrates away, it causes altered hormonal states and electrolyte imbalances that are responsible for the associated symptoms. The basic symptoms include headache, nausea, upset stomach, sleepiness, fatigue, abdominal cramps, diarrhea, and lack of mental clarity, or what is commonly referred to as "brain fog."

FACT

Carbohydrate addiction is a real thing. Some research shows that carbohydrates activate certain stimuli in the brain that can be dependence-forming and cause addiction. Carbohydrate addicts have uncontrollable cravings for carbohydrates, and when they do eat them, they tend to binge. In a carbohydrate addict, the removal of carbohydrates can cause withdrawal symptoms, such as dizziness and irritability, and intense cravings.

The duration of symptoms varies—it depends on you as an individual, but typically a "keto flu" lasts anywhere from a couple of days to a week. In rare cases, it can last up to two weeks. Some of the symptoms of the "keto flu" are associated with dehydration, because in the beginning stages of ketosis you lose a lot of water weight. With that lost fluid, you also lose electrolytes. You can replenish these electrolytes by drinking enhanced waters (but make sure they are not sweetened) and drinking lots of homemade bone broth. This may help lessen the severity of the symptoms.

Bad Breath

Unfortunately, bad breath is another early sign that you're in ketosis. When you're in ketosis, your body creates acetone as a waste product. Some of this acetone is released in your breath, giving it a fruity or ammonia-like quality. You can combat bad breath by chewing on fresh mint leaves and drinking plenty of water, since bad breath is also associated with dehydration.

Decreased Appetite and Nausea

As your body adapts to a ketogenic diet, you may have a decreased appetite. This is because you're providing your body with plenty of fat and protein, which are both highly satiating, and not a lot of carbohydrates. The nausea associated with "keto flu" can also decrease your appetite. When you reach this stage, it's important that you eat even if you feel like you aren't hungry. You want to make sure your body is getting enough calories and nutrients, especially in this time of transition.

Increased Energy

When the fog begins to clear and your body starts to become keto-adapted, the uncomfortable symptoms you were feeling will dissipate and you'll begin to see the benefits of following a ketogenic diet. One of the first beneficial signs many people experience is an increase in energy. When your body breaks down fat instead of carbohydrates, more energy is produced gram for gram, leaving you feeling alert and energized.

Improved Focus and Mental Clarity

Many mental issues, such as brain fog and problems with memory, are caused by what is called neurotoxicity, the exposure of the nervous system to toxic substances. For the brain, exposure to too much glucose can result in neurotoxicity. When you reduce the supply of glucose in your body and your brain starts to use ketones as fuel, the toxicity levels diminish. As a result, you may be able to think more clearly, focus better, and have better memory recall.

Other Possible Signs

Other possible signs of ketosis include:

- Cold hands and feet
- Increased urinary frequency
- Difficulty sleeping
- Metallic taste in the mouth
- Dry mouth
- Increased thirst

Measurable Ketones

Your body is pretty good at letting you know when you're in ketosis without any testing, but if you want to be absolutely sure, you can test your ketone levels with urine strips or a blood meter. Urine strips allow you to easily test for the presence of ketones in your urine, while blood meters can test for ketones with a small blood sample from a prick in your finger. These testing methods tend to be more reliable than just trusting the presence of symptoms, and if you really want to know if you're producing ketones, they're a great way to find out, but sometimes they can be inaccurate.

Although these signs are common among many people who follow a ketogenic diet, your experience may be different. Every body is unique, so it's impossible to say exactly what your personal experience will be. Keep in mind that in the early stages of ketosis, your symptoms may be unpleasant, but as your body adapts, you will begin to experience the benefits of following a ketogenic diet plan.

Managing Uncomfortable Symptoms

The initial symptoms of a ketogenic diet are uncomfortable, but if you choose to ride it out, you can rest assured that in time, they will go away. If the thought of being uncomfortable is really too much to bear, there are a few things you can try to help decrease the chances of experiencing symptoms, or at least lessen their severity.

Start Slowly

Like anything else, symptoms tend to be the worst when you transition to a ketogenic diet cold turkey. If you've been following a high-carbohydrate, low-fat diet for years—even decades—abruptly asking your body to run on fat instead is like a slap in the face. Instead of jumping right into a ketogenic diet, transition slowly.

Start by gradually eliminating non-nutritive carbohydrate sources, such as soda, desserts, sugary snacks, pasta, and pizza, over a period of a few weeks. As you eliminate these carbohydrate sources, increase the amount of fats you eat—coconut, avocado, and cheese, for example. When you've gotten used to the general principles of the diet, start tracking specific numbers and macronutrient ratios.

Snack Regularly

Eating a high-fat, moderate-protein snack, such as a fat bomb (see recipes in Chapter 15)—a snack that serves as concentrated source of healthy fats—may help ease certain symptoms, including headache and irritability. When you're first starting a ketogenic diet, make sure to snack regularly to keep yourself from getting too hungry. You may also consider protein shakes with amino acid supplements, which can help soften the transition. Just make sure these shakes are low in carbohydrates and don't contain a bevy of artificial ingredients.

Drink Water

Many of the symptoms, such as bad breath, are associated with being dehydrated. Drink plenty of water while you're transitioning and for the entire duration of your ketogenic diet. In addition to keeping you hydrated, water dilutes the ketone bodies, which can help alleviate symptoms.

CHAPTER 2

All about Fat

If you're one of the people who followed a low-fat diet and failed to lose weight, or failed to see any other major health improvements, don't worry; you're in the company of millions. When the popularity of the low-fat diet surged, many followers found themselves gaining more weight. Removing fat from your diet was supposed to make you thinner and healthier, but it did just the opposite. When people started replacing fats with carbohydrates and low-fat alternatives, the incidences of diabetes and obesity began to skyrocket. Could the beloved low-fat diet be to blame? Absolutely.

Low-Fat Diet Myths

If you're still on the low-fat diet train, read this next sentence carefully and really let it sink in: Fat is not your enemy; sugar is. And that applies to all forms of sugar, not only the granulated stuff that you put in your coffee in the morning. Sure, the sugar in fruit is packaged with vitamin C, potassium, fiber, and other valuable nutrients, which makes it a far superior choice over regular old sugar, but overdoing it can actually hinder weight loss efforts and set you up for other health problems. But before delving too deeply into sugar, it's important to spend some time debunking the myths that have surrounded the word "fat" for years.

FACT

As the low-fat diet began to gain popularity, there was also an increase in the availability of low-fat food items, such as cookies and candy bars. To create these items, manufacturers removed fat and replaced it with sugar to keep it palatable so consumers would continue to buy the product. These packaged food items were lower in fat, but they were higher in sugar and contained the same, if not more, calories.

Eating Fat Makes You Fat

On the surface, the theory that eating fat makes you fat seems like a no-brainer. Of the three macronutrients—protein, carbohydrates, and fat—fat contains the most calories per gram. Protein and carbohydrates have 4 calories per gram, while fat contains more than twice that at 9 calories per gram. It would make sense that if you cut out fat or replace fat with protein or carbohydrates at each meal, you would be saving yourself a ton of calories throughout the course of the day. While technically you would save on calories, it doesn't lead to sustainable weight loss.

In order to understand why fat doesn't make you fat, you have to understand how you gain weight in the first place. The simple explanation is this: You start thinking about food and your body secretes insulin in response. The insulin triggers a response that tells your body to store fatty acids instead of using them for energy, so you get hungry. When you get hungry, you eat. If you're on a low-fat diet, your lunch may consist of two slices of whole-wheat toast with a couple of slices of turkey—no cheese, no mayo—and an apple on the side. If you've subscribed to the low-fat diet theory, this seems like a healthy meal, but in reality, it's loaded with carbohydrates that pass through your digestive system quickly, causing significant spikes in blood sugar, and has virtually no fat.

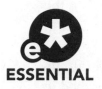

ESSENTIAL

Carbohydrates are a fast-acting source of energy for your body, but they don't do a lot to fill you up. Even carbohydrates that are loaded with fiber are far less satiating than either protein or fat. If you want your meal to be truly satisfying, make sure it contains plenty of fat.

Your body quickly breaks down your high-carbohydrate meal, which sends a rush of glucose into your bloodstream. Your body responds to this glucose by secreting more insulin, which carries the glucose out of your blood and into your cells. Once the glucose levels drop, you get hungry again, your body secretes more insulin, and the cycle starts over.

Now here's where you'll want to pay close attention. Your body's main regulator of fat metabolism is insulin. Insulin controls lipoprotein lipase, or LPL, an enzyme that pulls fat into your cells. The higher your insulin levels, the more fat LPL pulls into your cells. Translation: when insulin levels increase, you store fat. When insulin levels drop, you burn fat for energy. The main thing that affects insulin levels is carbohydrates, not fat. So when you eat a lot of carbohydrates, your insulin levels increase, which increases your LPL levels, which increases your storage of fat.

It's important to remember that overdoing it on any of the nutrients will lead to weight gain. Regularly exceeding your calorie needs will cause weight gain regardless of whether you do it with carbohydrates, protein, or fat—but fat is not the major culprit when it comes to weight gain.

Cholesterol Causes Heart Disease

The cholesterol you eat actually has very little impact on your blood cholesterol levels for two reasons. The first reason is that your body doesn't absorb dietary cholesterol very efficiently. Most of the cholesterol you eat goes right through your digestive tract and never even enters your bloodstream. The second reason is that the amount of cholesterol in your blood is tightly controlled by your body. When you eat a lot of dietary cholesterol, your body shuts down its own production of cholesterol to compensate. There is a percentage of the population, however, that is hypersensitive to dietary cholesterol. For these people—about 25 percent of the population—dietary cholesterol does cause modest increases in both LDL (low-density lipoprotein) and HDL (high-density lipoprotein) levels, but even so, the increased cholesterol levels do not increase the risk of heart disease. In fact, both the Framingham Heart Study and the Honolulu Heart Program Study both found the opposite to be true: low cholesterol levels were actually associated with increased risk of death. A separate study published in the *Journal of the American Medical Association* reported findings that neither high LDL ("bad" cholesterol) levels nor low HDL ("good" cholesterol) levels were important risk factors for death from coronary artery disease or heart attack.

FACT

Most of the cholesterol in your blood (75 percent) is actually made in your body. Only 25 percent comes from the food you eat. If you followed a completely cholesterol-free diet, your body would compensate by increasing its cholesterol production by the liver to keep your blood levels steady. That's because your body needs cholesterol to survive.

Cholesterol is absolutely essential for your survival. This lipoprotein, as it is physiologically classified, performs three major functions. It makes up the bile acids that help you digest food; it allows the body to make vitamin D and other essential hormones such as estrogen and testosterone; and it is a component of the outer coating of every one of your cells. Without cholesterol, your body would literally crumble.

Now that's not to say that you should throw all caution out the window when it comes to cholesterol, but you need to pay attention to the right thing, and that's the size of the cholesterol particles in your bloodstream rather than the total numbers. Cholesterol comes in two forms: large particles that "bounce" off the arterial walls and small, dense particles that stick to the walls of your arteries and contribute to arterial blockage, which can eventually lead to heart disease. The problem is that so much focus is placed on the total numbers that many people fail to pay attention to cholesterol particle size.

According to Dr. Mark Hyman, a functional medicine doctor at the UltraWellness Center in Lenox, Massachusetts, it's not fat that causes the accumulation of small, dense cholesterol particles in your blood, it's sugar. And that's sugar in any form, including refined carbohydrates. Sugar decreases the amount of the large cholesterol particles in your blood, creates the small damaging cholesterol particles, increases triglyceride levels, and contributes to pre-diabetes.

Saturated Fat Causes Heart Disease

The other widespread belief is that eating saturated fat causes an increase in the amount of cholesterol in your blood, which in turn causes heart disease or increases your risk of heart disease. This theory was developed from some human and animal studies that were done decades ago. However, more recent research calls these theories into question.

ESSENTIAL

The idea that eating cholesterol causes heart disease is called the diet-heart hypothesis. The theory that high cholesterol levels in the blood cause heart disease is called the lipid hypothesis. Both of these hypotheses are so widely accepted that most healthcare professionals and consumers don't even question them, although more recent research has shown that cholesterol and heart disease may not be as interconnected as previously believed.

In 2010, the *American Journal of Clinical Nutrition* did a meta-analysis of several studies that investigated the relationship between saturated fat and heart disease and concluded that there is no significant evidence to make the claim that dietary saturated fat is associated with increased risk of coronary heart disease or cardiovascular disease, in general. In fact, several of the studies the journal investigated showed a positive inverse relationship, which means that a higher intake of saturated fat was actually associated with a lower incidence of heart disease.

Researchers went even further to suggest that more analysis be done to determine whether the nutrients that replaced saturated fat actually had more of an influence on the risk of developing heart disease. After all, the nutrient that was used to replace saturated fat on low-fat diets was carbohydrates.

Why Fat Is Your Friend

Fat is an integral part of every cell in your body. This macronutrient is a major component of your cell membranes, which hold each cell together. Every single cell in your body, from the cells in your brain to the cells in your heart to the cells in your lungs, is dependent on fat for survival. Fat is especially important for your brain, which is made up of 60 percent fat and cholesterol.

Fat and cholesterol are used as building blocks for many hormones, which help regulate metabolism, control growth and development, and maintain bone and muscle mass, among many other things. Fat is vital for proper immune function, helps regulate body temperature, and serves as a source of protection for your major organs. Fat surrounds all of your vital organs to provide a sort of cushion for protection against falls and trauma. Fat also helps boost metabolic function and plays a role in keeping you lean.

Fat is an essential nutrient. This means that you need to ingest it through the foods you eat because the body cannot make what it needs on its own. Fat is composed of individual molecules called fatty acids. Two of these fatty acids, omega-3 fatty acids and omega-6 fatty acids, are absolutely essential for good health. Omega-3 fatty acids play a crucial role in brain function and growth and development, while omega-6 fatty acids help regulate metabolism and maintain bone health. Fat also allows you to absorb and digest other essential nutrients, such as vitamins A, D, E, and K and beta-carotene. Without enough fat in your diet, you wouldn't be able to absorb any of these nutrients and you would eventually develop nutritional deficiencies.

As if that weren't enough, fat is a major source of energy for your body. The fact that each gram of fat contains 9 calories is actually a good thing. This makes it a compact source of energy that your body can use easily and efficiently. Unlike with carbohydrates, which your body can only store in limited amounts, your body has an unlimited ability to store fat for later use. When food intake falls short, as between meals or while you're sleeping, your body calls on its fat reservoirs for energy. This physiological process is what the entire ketogenic diet is based on.

Your body needs a continuous source of energy to maintain its functions. The body's preferred source of energy, because it's fast-acting and easily accessible, is glucose, which comes from carbohydrates. When you give your body access to glucose, it stores fat in your fat cells for later use. When you deprive the body of glucose, it turns to fat for energy.

Reducing Body Fat

Now that you know what causes your body to store fat, the obvious next question is, how do you use that knowledge to help reduce your body fat? The quick answer, and one that may seem counterintuitive at this point, is to eat more fat, but it's not that simple. You can't simply add fat to a diet that's full of carbohydrates and loaded with protein and expect the weight to fall off. You have to make a strategic plan to follow a diet that allows you to eat a significant amount of fat while also limiting carbohydrate intake and eating a moderate amount of protein. In other words: a ketogenic diet.

FACT

Researchers at the Karolinska Institute in Stockholm, Sweden, found that the number of fat cells you have as an adult remains the same no matter how much weight you lose. When you lose weight, the number of fat cells doesn't actually decrease; the cells just shrink in size, essentially taking up less room and making you look leaner.

The Importance of a Healthy Body Fat Level

Fat is important, there's no doubt about that, but too much on your body can be bad for your health. Having excess body fat increases your risk of various health problems, including:

- Type 2 diabetes
- Heart disease
- Gallstones
- Sleep apnea
- Certain types of cancers
- High blood pressure
- Stroke
- Osteoarthritis
- Fatty liver disease
- Infertility
- Kidney disease
- Gestational diabetes

Reducing the amount of fat you carry on your body can help reduce your risk of developing these chronic conditions, even if you have a family history of them.

Improving Your Blood Sugar and Insulin Levels

A major component to keeping yourself healthy, or improving any current health problems, is regulating your blood sugar and insulin levels. Imbalances in blood sugar and insulin are significant factors in the rapidly growing epidemic in diabetes in both children and adults.

Insulin Resistance and Diabetes

You already know that insulin is responsible for bringing the glucose from your bloodstream into your cells so that your body can use it as energy, but insulin also stimulates your liver and muscles to store excess glucose, which is called glycogen, for later use. In a healthy person, insulin and glucose do their jobs effectively and efficiently, and as a result, both insulin and glucose levels remain within a certain healthy range.

Insulin resistance is a condition in which the pancreas produces enough insulin, but the body does not use it effectively. When you're repeatedly exposed to high levels of insulin, your cells begin to say, "No, thank you" and start building up a resistance to insulin. When insulin, which carries glucose on its back, can't enter the cells, glucose remains in the bloodstream as well. This signals the pancreas to release even more insulin, which only exacerbates the cycle. While your body may be able to sustain this added stress for a certain period of time, eventually the pancreas gives up and insulin production decreases or stops altogether.

ALERT

Many people aren't aware that they have insulin resistance until they are officially diagnosed with pre-diabetes or type 2 diabetes. Early warning signs of insulin resistance include fatigue, energy crashes, carbohydrate cravings, and weight gain around the midsection. If you experience any of these warning signs, it may be beneficial to have your insulin and glucose levels tested.

Without insulin, glucose can't enter the cells, so it stays in the bloodstream, wreaking havoc on your system. This is the point when many people are diagnosed with pre-diabetes or type 2 diabetes. Elevated glucose levels also contribute to obesity, high blood pressure, heart disease, certain types of cancer, and neurodegenerative disorders such as Alzheimer's disease.

What's Carbs Got to Do with It?

When you eat carbohydrates, your body breaks them down into glucose. The rate at which this happens differs depending on the type of carbohydrates you're eating, but eventually, all carbohydrates, with the exception of fiber, become glucose. When glucose enters your bloodstream, it triggers the release of insulin, as you already know. Constantly bombarding your body with carbohydrates and refined sugars increases glucose and insulin levels dramatically, increasing your risk of developing insulin resistance and the other resulting health problems. The goal is to avoid surges and crashes in glucose and insulin and to keep your levels consistent and steady throughout the day. When you do this, your body is better able to handle both glucose and insulin over the long-term.

How Fat Can Help

Unlike carbohydrates and refined sugars, eating fat doesn't cause a dramatic spike in glucose or insulin levels. When you turn your body from burning glucose for fuel to burning fat for fuel, which is the basis of the ketogenic diet, you help stabilize your glucose and insulin levels, which decreases your chances of developing insulin resistance.

Feeling Satisfied While Losing Weight

One of the biggest complaints you'll hear from dieters on a weight-loss program is that they don't feel satisfied. They're always hungry or the food just isn't good. This is where most diets fail. If you're always hungry on a diet, what are the chances that you're going to be able to stick to it long-term? Probably close to zero. No one wants to be hungry all the time. On the other hand, consistently eating foods that lack any flavor and always leave you wanting more is a recipe for disaster. At some point, your cravings for delicious, satiating foods are going to triumph over your determination to lose weight and you're going to give in to temptation—and probably in a big way. Feelings of deprivation are one of the biggest causes of eventual binges. This is where fat shines.

FACT

Foods with a high fat content tend to taste so good because many different flavors dissolve in fats. Butter especially works as an excellent carrier for a wide variety of flavors, including spices, vanilla, and other fat-soluble ingredients. The human body is also genetically programmed to seek out high-energy foods. Because of this, fatty foods are inherently perceived as more flavorful.

Of the three macronutrients, fat is the most satiating. Sure it's the calorie-densest, too, but it helps you fill up faster and keeps you full longer, which means that you're likely to take in fewer calories over the long term and you're less prone to uncontrollable binges. When you cut fat out of your diet, it's hard to reach that point when you really feel satisfied. This is why people on low-fat diets complain of being hungry all the time. Fat also adds a ton of flavor to food, so when you eat fat you're actually enjoying the food you're eating, which makes you more likely to stick to your diet plan. Sounds like a no-brainer, right?

CHAPTER 3

Ketogenic Diet Basics

Now that you have a full understanding of how the body obtains energy and what ketosis is (a state during which your body relies on fat for energy instead of carbohydrates), it's time to put all that information to good use. As the name implies, the ketogenic diet is a diet plan that puts your body's innate intelligence to work by forcing your body to enter into a state of ketosis. Your body already instinctively knows how to do this when you don't eat carbohydrates, but the point of the ketogenic diet is to force it to happen and keep it going for as long as you want. If you're interested in starting a ketogenic diet, a qualified nutrition or healthcare professional can help you get started.

What Is the Ketogenic Diet?

The ketogenic diet encourages you to get most of your calories from fat and severely restrict carbohydrates. Unlike a typical low-carbohydrate diet, the ketogenic diet is not a high-protein diet. Instead, it's a high-fat, moderate-protein, and low-carbohydrate diet. Although your exact macronutrient ratio will differ based on your individual needs, a typical nutritional ketogenic diet looks something like this:

- Fat: 60 to 75 percent of calories
- Protein: 15 to 30 percent of calories
- Carbohydrates: 5 to 10 percent of calories

These are just general guidelines, but most people on a successful ketogenic diet fall somewhere in this range. In order to figure what you should be eating, you'll have to calculate your individual macronutrient ratios. As your diet progresses and your body begins to change, you may have to recalculate these numbers and make the proper adjustments to your diet plan.

Calculating Your Macronutrient Ratio

The first thing you need to do to calculate your macronutrient ratio is figure out how many calories you should be eating. There are several online calculators that can calculate this number for you, but to do it yourself, you can use a method called the Mifflin-St Jeor formula, which looks like this:

- Men: $10 \times$ weight (kg) $+ 6.25 \times$ height (cm) $- 5 \times$ age (y) $+ 5$
- Women: $10 \times$ weight (kg) $+ 6.25 \times$ height (cm) $- 5 \times$ age (y) $- 161$

To make this explanation easier, let's try using the equation with a 30-year-old, 160-pound (72.7 kg) woman who is 5 feet 5 inches (165.1 cm) tall. When you plug this woman's statistics into the Mifflin-St Jeor formula, you can see that she should be eating 1,448 calories per day. Now you'll use the estimated macronutrient percentages to calculate how much of each nutrient she needs to consume in order to follow a successful ketogenic diet plan.

Carbohydrates

On a ketogenic diet, carbohydrates should provide only 5 to 10 percent of the calories you consume. Many ketogenic dieters stay at the low end of 5 percent, but the exact amount you need depends on your body. Unfortunately, there is no one-size-fits-all approach to this, so you'll have to do a little trial and error. You can pick a percentage that feels right for you and try that out for a couple of weeks. If you don't see the results you want, you'll have to adjust your nutrient ratios and calculate them again. Getting 7 percent of your calories from carbohydrates is a good place to start.

To calculate how many grams of carbohydrates this is, multiply 7 percent by the total number of calories, which, in the earlier example, is 1,448, and then divide by 4 (since carbohydrates contain 4 calories per gram). The number you're left with is the amount of carbohydrates in grams you should eat per day. In this example, the number is 25 grams.

Total Carbohydrates versus Net Carbohydrates

When counting carbohydrates on a ketogenic diet plan, you want to pay attention to net carbohydrates, not total carbohydrates. Net carbohydrates are the amount of carbohydrates left over after you subtract grams of fiber from total grams of carbohydrates. If a particular food contains 10 grams of carbohydrates, but 7 grams come from fiber, the total number of net carbohydrates is 3 grams. You count the 3 grams toward your daily total, rather than the 10 grams.

Fat

After you've calculated carbohydrates, move on to fat. Again, the exact amount you'll need depends on you as an individual, but consuming 75 percent of your calories from fat is a good place to start. To figure out the amount of fat you need in grams, multiply the amount of calories you need (in this example, 1,448) by 75 percent and then divide by 9 (since fat contains 9 calories per gram). The number you're left with is the total grams of fat you need for the day. In this example, it's 121 grams.

Protein

Once you've calculated carbohydrates and fat, protein is easy. The remainder of your calories, which equates to 18 percent, should come from protein. To figure out this number in grams, multiply the total number of calories by 18 percent and then divide by 4 (since protein contains 4 calories per gram). The number you're left with is the total grams of protein you need for the day. In this example, it's 65 grams.

ESSENTIAL

As your body changes, your macronutrient ranges may also change. When following a ketogenic diet, it's beneficial to recalculate your nutrient needs regularly—about once per month. If your needs change, adjust your diet accordingly.

Foods to Eat and Avoid

When following a ketogenic diet, some foods are strictly off-limits, while others fall into a sort of gray area. Regardless of whether foods are "allowed," you still have to make sure that you're staying within your macronutrient ratios. Just because a food is technically allowed doesn't mean you can eat as much of it as you want. Use these recommendations as a guideline, but always make sure that you're staying within your calculated macronutrient ratios.

A Word on Quality

The quality of your food matters, especially when it comes to fat and protein sources. Ideally, you want to choose meats that are organic, grass-fed, and pasture-raised. Eggs should come from your local farmer or from pasture-raised hens whenever possible. Choose grass-fed butter and organic creams, cheese, fruits, and vegetables. Eating conventional foods won't prevent you from entering a ketogenic state, but high-quality foods are better for your body in general. After all, you are what you eat. Do your best to get the highest quality food you can find and/or afford.

Fats and Oils

Fats and oils provide the basis of your ketogenic diet, so you'll want to make sure you're eating plenty of them. The ketogenic diet is not just a fat free-for-all, though. While following a ketogenic diet, there are certain fats that are better for you than others, although which ones fall into which category may surprise you. On the ketogenic diet, you should eat plenty of saturated fats in the form of meat, poultry, eggs, butter, and coconut; mono-unsaturated fats, such as olive oil, nuts, nut butters, and avocado; and natural polyunsaturated fats, such as tuna, salmon, and mackerel. Avoid highly processed polyunsaturated fats, such as canola oil, vegetable oil, and soybean oil. Homemade Mayonnaise is also an easy way to add a dose of fat to every meal.

Proteins

Many of the fat sources mentioned previously—meat, poultry, eggs, butter, nuts, nut butters, and fish—are also loaded with protein and should be your main protein sources when following a ketogenic diet. Bacon and sausage are other sources of protein that also provide a significant dose of fat. When eating protein make sure to stay within your recommended grams for the day, since your body turns excess protein into glucose, which can kick you out of ketosis.

Fruits and Vegetables

When following a ketogenic diet, most fruits fall onto the "do not eat" list. Even though the sugars in fruit are natural sugars, they still raise your blood glucose levels significantly and can kick you out of ketosis. There's not a hard rule that fruit isn't allowed on a ketogenic diet, but you do need to limit your intake. When you do eat fruit, choose fruits that are high in fiber and lower in carbohydrates, such as berries, and limit your portions.

Vegetables are extremely important on a ketogenic diet. They provide the vitamins and minerals that you need to stay healthy and help fill you up without contributing a lot of calories to your day. You do have to be choosy about which vegetables you eat, though, since some are loaded with carbohydrates and do not have a place on a ketogenic diet.

As a general rule, choose dark green or leafy green vegetables, such as spinach, broccoli, cucumbers, green beans, lettuce, and asparagus. Cauliflower and mushrooms are also good choices for a ketogenic diet. Avoid starchy vegetables, including white potatoes, sweet potatoes, yams, and corn.

Dairy

Full-fat dairy products are a staple on the ketogenic diet. Use butter, heavy cream, sour cream, cream cheese, hard cheese, and cottage cheese to help meet your fat needs. Avoid low-fat dairy products and flavored dairy products, such as fruity yogurt. Flavored yogurt is full of sugar; serving for serving, some versions contain as much sugar and carbohydrates as soda.

Beverages

As with any diet plan, when it comes to beverages, water is your best bet. Make sure to drink at least half of your body weight in ounces. Coffee and tea are also permitted on a ketogenic diet, but they must be unsweetened or sweetened with an approved sweetener, such as stevia or erythritol. Avoid sodas, flavored waters, sweetened teas, sweetened lemonade, and fruit juices. You can infuse plain water with fresh herbs, such as mint or basil, to give yourself a little variety.

Grains and Sugars

Avoid grains and sugars in all of their forms on the ketogenic diet. Grains include wheat, barley, rice, rye, sorghum, and anything made from these products. That means no breads, no pasta, no crackers, and no rice. Sugar, and anything that contains sugar, is also not allowed on a ketogenic diet. This includes white sugar, brown sugar, honey, maple syrup, corn syrup, and brown rice syrup. There are many names for sugar on ingredient lists; it's extremely beneficial to familiarize yourself with these names so you'll know when a product contains sugar in any form.

Intermittent Fasting on the Ketogenic Diet

Intermittent fasting has recently gained popularity as a supplement to your diet plan. The basic premise behind intermittent fasting is that you can overcome a weight-loss plateau by completely restricting all food intake for a certain period of time. It is believed that when you deny your body food, your body has to break down stored fat for energy instead. There are a few different types of intermittent fasting.

The first is simply skipping meals. Many people who decide to incorporate intermittent fasting into their ketogenic diet plan stop eating after dinner and skip over breakfast to extend the period of time that the body goes without food. Another form of intermittent fasting is giving yourself certain "eating windows." An eating window is a period of time that you allow yourself to eat; the rest of the time you spend fasting. A typical eating window is between 4 and 7 hours, so you may decide that you'll eat all of your meals between 2 P.M. and 7 P.M. and then you don't eat outside of these windows. The last, and most extreme, form of intermittent fasting is to completely avoid food for 24 to 48 hours. This is an extreme form of intermittent fasting and is not recommended. Some people incorporate intermittent fasting every day and others do it once or twice per week.

ESSENTIAL

Although there are anecdotal reports that intermittent fasting can help ketogenic dieters overcome a weight-loss plateau, this has not yet been scientifically proven. If you do decide to incorporate intermittent fasting into your ketogenic diet, you may have to play around with it to judge whether or not it works for you. Consult a qualified health-care professional before incorporating intermittent fasting into your eating routine, especially if you have an existing medical condition.

Starting a Ketogenic Diet

If you're used to following a standard American diet—one in which most of your calories come from carbohydrates—a ketogenic diet is a major change. You have two choices: jump into it cold turkey or slowly wean yourself off carbohydrates, increasing your fat intake until your macronu-trient ratios fall within your goal. When you go into it cold turkey, you're more likely to experience unpleasant carbohydrate withdrawal symptoms, so easing into it slowly is often the best bet for success.

Carbohydrate Guides

Carbohydrate guides are a helpful tool to use with the ketogenic diet, especially when you're just starting out. Many books are available that pro-vide a list of foods and their carbohydrate count (as well as their calorie, protein, and fat content). Some of these books categorize foods into high-carbohydrate, medium-carbohydrate, and low-carbohydrate lists. There are also several mobile apps that do the same thing.

Whatever method you choose, make sure you have your carbohydrate guide handy when you're food shopping so you can double-check what foods are allowed on the diet and which foods aren't. As you get the hang of the diet, you won't need to check every single food before you purchase it, but it's still handy to have the guides easily accessible for those once-in-a-while foods that you're unsure about.

Prepare Your Kitchen

Once you've made the decision to start a ketogenic diet, you need to pre-pare your kitchen. This is a two-part process: you'll need to remove off-plan foods and stock your refrigerator and pantry with the essentials. If you live alone or with others who are also following a ketogenic diet, removing off-plan foods is simple. Go through your pantry and refrigerator and take out all the foods that don't fit into your diet plan. Don't forget to check the labels on your spices and dried herbs. Sometimes these contain sugar or other artificial ingredients that don't belong on a ketogenic diet. Donate unopened items to your local food pantry and toss the open ones in the trash.

If you're the only one in your household starting a ketogenic diet, this removal process is a little more complicated. Instead of donating or throw-ing out foods that are off-plan, divide the pantry up. If possible, put all ketogenic-approved foods in a separate cabinet and make it a point to only go in there and not even look in the off-plan cabinet. Dividing up the fridge might be even more difficult than dividing the pantry, but do the best you can to separate what you can eat from what you can't.

The second part of preparing your kitchen is to stock up on all the essentials. It's imperative that you always have foods on hand that you can eat. If you don't, you're more likely to get to the point of being so hungry that you'll eat anything. Familiarize yourself with the essentials listed in Appendix A and keep your kitchen stocked with them at all times.

Ease Into It

When you're excited about starting a new diet, it's tempting to jump right in, but your body will thank you if you ease it into the ketogenic diet slowly. Doing so will lessen the severity of any of the "keto flu" symptoms you might experience and make the transition a little easier. Give yourself about three to four weeks from the time you commit to following a ketogenic diet to the day you actually start it 100 percent.

ALERT

Although artificially sweetened beverages are allowed on a ketogenic diet because they don't contain any carbohydrates, try to avoid them. Some research shows that even though artificial sweeteners don't contain any calories, they can contribute to weight gain. Plus, part of the goal is to try to get rid of your sweet tooth, and drinking sweetened beverages won't help you do that.

During the first week, cut out all sugary beverages. This includes soda, lemonade, sweetened teas, and flavored waters. If you put sugar in your coffee, scale back—use one teaspoon instead of two. After one week of this, remove all desserts and sugary snacks from your diet, including candy, cookies, cakes, muffins, chocolates, and ice cream. Get in the habit of not having dessert after dinner. You want to train your body to stop craving sweets and one way to do this is to cut them out completely, especially while you're transitioning to a ketogenic diet. On your third week, cut out starchy carbohydrates such as pasta, pizza, bread, crackers, rolls, and potatoes. At this point, you may have already started to lose weight.

When you start week 4, you'll be ready to officially start your ketogenic diet. This is when you should start tracking your macronutrients to make sure you're staying within the correct ratios. Limiting carbohydrates is important, but it's not the only goal; make sure you're also eating plenty of fat and moderate amounts of protein.

ESSENTIAL

Years ago, unless you had the fancy, expensive software that nutritionists use, the only way to track your macronutrients was by looking up each food item, writing down its carbohydrate, protein, and fat content, and adding it all up. Nowadays, there are several apps that you can download on your phone that will do the work for you. Make your life easier by downloading one of these apps—a popular one is MyFitnessPal—and tracking everything you eat.

Stay Hydrated and Replenish Electrolytes

Staying hydrated is always important, but it's especially vital when you're starting a ketogenic diet. It's not only about drinking water; you also want to replenish your electrolytes. When you start a ketogenic diet, you initially lose water, which takes electrolytes such as sodium and potassium with it. Aim to drink the equivalent of at least half your body weight in ounces. This means that, for example, if you're 180 pounds, you'll want to drink at least 90 ounces of water a day.

You can replenish your electrolytes by drinking a cup of homemade bone broth every day, adding salt to your foods, and drinking waters that are enhanced with electrolytes. Just make sure that the enhanced waters are unflavored, as the flavored waters often contain a lot of sugar and other artificial ingredients.

ESSENTIAL

The soup stocks and broths that you get at the store are a lot different from the bone broth you make at home. To make an electrolyte-rich bone broth, get some high-quality soup bones from your local farmer or butcher. Put these bones in a pot and add enough water to just cover them. Add some salt and pepper, and some bay leaves if you prefer, and let the broth simmer for 12 to 24 hours.

Planning Meals for Long-Term Success

Planning your meals is vital to your long-term success on a ketogenic diet. There is a popular quote, most often credited to Benjamin Franklin, that goes something like this: "When you fail to plan, you plan to fail." It's true. The best way to ensure success is to plan your weekly meals, prepare meals in advance, and always make sure you have ketogenic-approved snacks on hand.

Meal Planning

Take one night a week and write out everything you will eat all week. Plan your meals and your snacks and then compile a grocery list for what you'll need in order to execute these meals and snacks. You may choose to make your meal-planning day your shopping day, as well. Get everything you need in one swoop and then don't stray from your plan.

Meal Prep

Once you know what you're going to eat all week, you may decide that you want to cook each meal individually, or you may decide that spending a few hours prepping your meals makes more sense for you. If you choose the latter, pick a day when you don't have any other commitments and spend a few hours in the kitchen preparing your meals for the entire week. You can make a quiche, a couple of ketogenic-friendly casseroles, and a big pot of soup. Divide each meal into to-go containers and store them in the refrigerator so that they're ready to go when you are.

Being Prepared

When you're on a specialized diet such as the ketogenic one, there is really no such thing as convenience foods. You have to be prepared at all times. You might have to take meals and snacks with you everywhere you go, but it's a small price to pay for the way you'll feel. Pack a lunch every day and keep nonperishable snacks, like fat bombs, coconut shavings, nuts, and seeds in your car, in your desk at work, and in your purse or briefcase.

Don't Make It Complicated

It's tempting to want to create elaborate meal plans that feature a new gourmet entrée each night, but for most people that's just not realistic. You have to make sure that your new diet plan can fit into your lifestyle, otherwise you won't be able to stick to it. Keep things simple by eating the same thing for breakfast three times a week and using leftovers from dinner for the next day's lunch. You can double or triple recipes to prepare meals in bulk and then freeze them for another day when you don't have the time to cook.

Starting a new diet is not easy; it takes dedication and preparation. You'll have to do some fine-tuning and rearranging to figure out what works for you, but once you get the hang of it, it will become second nature.

CHAPTER 4

Medical Applications

Many people successfully use the ketogenic diet to lose weight or boost energy. Ketogenic dieters also experience mental clarity and improved focus and memory, but the benefits don't stop there. The ketogenic diet has been shown to be an effective therapy for several medical conditions, especially those that involve disruptions in nerve activity in the brain. For many of these conditions, researchers aren't entirely sure why the ketogenic diet works; they just know that it can.

The Ketogenic Diet for Epilepsy

Seizures come in many forms. They may be characterized by violent shaking or simply staring off into space for an extended period of time. A seizure occurs when the nerve cell activity in the brain is disrupted for any particular reason. Those who experience recurrent seizures are often given a diagnosis of epilepsy. Epilepsy is not a disease, but rather the name of a group of neurological disorders characterized by recurring seizures without a known cause.

FACT

Approximately 10 percent of people will have a seizure at some point in their lifetime. Of those 10 percent, only 30 percent will have a second seizure. When the seizures occur frequently, and with no known underlying cause, it's called epilepsy.

The condition affects approximately 65 million people in the world. Currently, there are many medications available to help treat epilepsy, but approximately 30 percent of people with epilepsy don't respond to these medications. Some epileptic individuals may even benefit from surgery, but one of the oldest, and least invasive, epileptic treatment therapies is the ketogenic diet. Researchers aren't entirely sure how a ketogenic diet helps epilepsy, but research shows that the diet may elicit biochemical changes that prevent and eliminate short-circuits in the brain's signaling system that are responsible for the seizures.

The History of the Ketogenic Diet for Seizures

According to a report in the medical journal *Epilepsia*, fasting-type diets have been used to treat seizures since as early as 500 B.C. The first modern use of starvation as a treatment for epilepsy occurred in 1911 when Dr. Guelpa and Dr. Marie, two physicians from Paris, treated twenty adults and children with epilepsy and found that their symptoms were less severe during periods of metabolic starvation. This research was crucial to the introduction of the ketogenic diet as a dietary therapy for epilepsy.

In 1921, Dr. Wilder, a physician from the Mayo Clinic, hypothesized that you could achieve the benefits of fasting through other means besides completely restricting food, which isn't sustainable for the long term. Dr. Wilder said that not only would the ketogenic diet be just as effective as fasting, but patients could follow the diet for a long period of time because it supplied most of the nutrients that the body needed.

A colleague of Dr. Wilder, Dr. Peterman, calculated the ratios of macronutrients and came up with a plan that allowed dieters 1 gram of protein per kilogram of body weight, 10–15 grams of net carbohydrates per day, and the remainder of their calories from fat. The diet was used as a major treatment therapy for epilepsy throughout the 1920s and 1930s with a high success rate. In a textbook published in 1972, Dr. Livingston from Johns Hopkins Hospital revealed the results of a ketogenic diet intervention that he tested on 1,000 children. He reported that 52 percent of participants had complete control of their seizures when following a ketogenic diet, while another 27 percent had a significant improvement in seizure control. At the time, physicians could find treatment plans and instructions on how to calculate meal plans in almost every textbook, but with a rise in availability of anti-seizure medications, the diet fell out of fashion. Medicine was thought to be the treatment of the future, so physicians and dietitians were no longer being trained in the diet and fewer children were placed on it. Currently, the ketogenic diet is still available as a treatment option for children with epilepsy in some select hospitals, but it's not as widely accepted or as well understood by physicians as it was in the past.

Who It Is For

As with any medical therapy, the ketogenic diet is not for everyone who experiences seizures. Doctors typically only recommend the ketogenic diet for children with difficult-to-control seizures (especially those with Lennox-Gastaut Syndrome). At the medical centers that still use the ketogenic diet, it's usually not implemented until at least two or three medications have been shown to be ineffective, and usually is recommended only for those who would not benefit from surgery.

Medical ketogenic diets for epilepsy should only be done under close supervision of a trained physician or nutrition professional. The diet is usually begun in a medical setting over a period of 3 or 4 days so that the child can be monitored closely. During this time, the physician monitors blood sugar levels and ketone levels and watches for any seizures.

Traditionally, the ketogenic diet has been used for children with difficult-to-treat myoclonic, atonic, and tonic-clonic seizures. Myoclonic seizures are brief, shock-like jerks in a muscle or a group of muscles. They typically don't last for more than a couple of seconds. Atonic seizures are characterized by a sudden loss in muscle strength. Someone having an atonic seizure may have a drooping eyelid or suddenly drop his head. A tonic-clonic seizure, which is also known as a grand mal seizure, is the type most people picture when they hear the word "seizure." Tonic-clonic seizures are characterized by a stiffening of the muscles followed by loss of consciousness. After the loss of consciousness comes rapid, rhythmic jerking of the muscles, especially in the arms and legs. A tonic-clonic seizure typically lasts 1 to 3 minutes.

The Diet Breakdown

A medical ketogenic diet is stricter than a nutritional ketogenic diet, with different macronutrient ratios. A typical medical ketogenic diet allows four times as much fat as protein and carbohydrate combined (called a 4:1 ratio), but some children are put on a 3:1 ratio, or a ketogenic diet that allows three times as much fat as protein and carbohydrate combined.

Because of its critical purpose, a medical ketogenic diet meal plan must be calculated by a trained dietitian or nutritionist and each food must be weighed out on a gram scale to make sure that the exact meal plan is being followed. Just one off-plan meal can throw a child out of ketosis and result in a seizure. A typical meal consists of a protein-rich food, a fruit or vegetable, and a source of fat, such as butter, heavy cream, or mayonnaise.

Assessing the Results

Because each person is unique, it's impossible to say with certainty whether or not the diet will help control seizures, but for those who do benefit, there is usually improvement in frequency and/or severity of seizures within the first ten weeks. Many children, especially those on more than one anti-seizure medication, are able to reduce the amount of medication they take. Some children are able to discontinue use of medication completely. If the diet is successful, it's typically used for a period of up to three years. If no improvement is seen within the first few months, your physician or nutritionist will usually recommend stopping the diet.

Several studies have shown that once children who have seen no improvement from multiple epileptic medications are put on a ketogenic diet, they experience significant results. Fifty percent of children on a ketogenic diet experience a 50 percent decrease in seizures; approximately 33 percent see an improvement of at least 90 percent; and 10 percent become seizure-free and are able to get off all medication.

Potential Side Effects

Although medical ketogenic diets are better tolerated than most medications, there is still a potential for side effects. The most common side effects are lack of weight gain, decreased growth, constipation, and kidney stones. Most of these side effects can be reversed without having to stop the diet. The physician or nutritionist who prescribed the diet will usually make adjustments to nutrient ratios or provide supplements that can help with side effects.

Alzheimer's Disease and Ketosis

Your brain contains 100 billion nerve cells. Each nerve cell is interconnected with millions of other nerve cells. These nerve cells communicate with each other to perform hundreds of functions, including remembering, thinking, and learning new things. Alzheimer's disease occurs when part of these nerve networks in the brain get destroyed. Researchers aren't exactly sure what causes the damage associated with Alzheimer's, but what they do know is that when the damage occurs, the nerve cells can no longer do their jobs.

Alzheimer's disease is the most common type of dementia—a general term that describes a decline in mental ability that is severe enough to interfere with day-to-day life. Someone with Alzheimer's disease usually experiences difficulty learning new information, memory loss, behavior changes, mood changes, disorientation, difficulty speaking and swallowing, trouble walking, and suspicions about family and friends. Healthcare professionals tend to agree that a combination of physical exercise, mental/social activity, and a healthy diet improve the brain health in those with Alzheimer's, but there is some disagreement about what actually constitutes a healthy diet for the condition.

FACT

Alzheimer's disease is the sixth leading cause of death in the United States and the fifth leading cause of death in Americans over the age of 65. Between the years 2000 and 2010, the number of deaths due to Alzheimer's increased by 68 percent.

Some health organizations recommend a diet that's low in all fat, especially saturated fat, and high in carbohydrates from fruits, vegetables, legumes, and whole grains, which is the complete opposite of a ketogenic diet. So what does the research say?

Recent studies have shown that Alzheimer's patients who follow a ketogenic diet may not only experience improvement in symptoms like cognition and memory, but may also experience a slowing of mental and physical decline. There is still some question as to why, but researchers believe it's because Alzheimer's disease is characterized by an inability of the brain to transport glucose across the blood-brain barrier. As a result, the cells in the brain become starved of sufficient glucose, which leads to neurodegeneration, or the dying of nerve cells in the brain. The solution then would be to supply the brain with a different form of energy: ketones.

A study published in 2009 in *Nutrition & Metabolism* reported that study participants with mild to moderate Alzheimer's disease who were given a ketogenic agent showed significant improvement in their symptoms. Another study published in 2010 reported that of 60 study participants with dementia who had medium-chain triglycerides (MCTs) added to their diets, 90 percent reported improvement in at least one group of symptoms, which included memory, thinking, social interaction, sleep, vision, and appetite.

Although there hasn't been enough specific research on ketogenic diets and Alzheimer's disease to make conclusive statements, the research to date is highly encouraging regarding the effect of MCTs and ketogenic agents on symptom improvement.

Can Ketosis Help Other Health Conditions?

Encouraged by the epilepsy and Alzheimer's study results, researchers have also been studying the effects of the ketogenic diet and resulting ketosis on other health conditions. Currently, there's not enough evidence to determine whether ketogenic diets should be a widely recommended part of the treatment for other health conditions, but the results of these preliminary studies have also been extremely positive.

Parkinson's Disease

Parkinson's disease belongs to a group of disorders called motor system disorders. In someone with Parkinson's, the dopamine-producing cells in the brain become destroyed and the production of the neurotransmitter dopamine declines. Dopamine controls muscular movement, permitting smooth and fluid motion. After 60 to 80 percent of the dopamine-producing cells in the brain are destroyed, the symptoms of Parkinson's, which include shaking, tremor, slowness of movement, stiffness, and trouble balancing, begin to appear.

FACT

In general, Parkinson's disease begins between the ages of 50 and 65. Approximately 1 percent of people in that age population are affected with the motor system disorder.

A study published in the medical journal *Neurology* reported that Parkinson's patients may see an improvement in symptoms when following a ketogenic diet. In the study, which didn't include a control group, Parkinson's patients were instructed to follow a ketogenic diet. After 28 days on the diet, all study participants reported moderate to very good improvements in symptoms.

Although it is not entirely clear how a ketogenic diet could help improve symptoms in people with Parkinson's disease, scientists theorize that the ketones may actually bypass the area in the brain that is damaged and provide much-needed energy to other areas in the brain. Another theory is that the ketones, which have an anti-inflammatory effect on the brain, may be able to mend damaged neurons.

Cancer

In 1923, a German biochemist named Otto Warburg suggested that cancer is caused by disruptions in normal metabolic processes that result in cancer cells taking up large amounts of energy in the form of glucose and converting it to lactate to produce energy. At the time, the hypothesis was highly controversial, but more recently, his theory, which is now deemed the Warburg effect, has gotten some attention.

Cancer cells feed on glucose, but unlike heart, muscle, and brain cells, which can adapt to obtaining energy from ketones, tumor cells can't get enough energy from ketones. As a result, researchers hypothesized that following a ketogenic diet may starve cancer cells of the glucose they need to survive and eventually they will die off. Like all good theories, this one was put to the test on several different occasions.

The first finding of the possibility of a ketogenic diet to help cancer was reported in 1995. Researchers put two brain cancer patients on a ketogenic diet that consisted of 60 percent MCTs (the fats that are found in high concentrations in coconuts), 10 percent other fats, 20 percent protein, and 10 percent carbohydrates. Both patients had aggressive brain tumors that were not responsive to traditional treatments and had been given a poor prognosis. After following the diet for a period of time, brain scans showed that the tumors started to shrink.

Another study published in 2007 reported that 16 brain cancer patients who were instructed to follow a ketogenic diet experienced improvement in symptoms and quality of life. A third study in 2010 reported that when a 65-year-old brain cancer patient was put on a restricted ketogenic diet, she reported cancer remission and absence of symptoms.

Although there isn't enough evidence to make conclusive statements about the potential role of the ketogenic diet in brain cancer treatment, the studies are promising.

Mitochondrial Disorders

Mitochondria are known as the energy powerhouses in your body. The mitochondria turn the nutrients from the food you eat into a compound called adenosine triphosphate, or ATP, which provides energy to all of your cells. In those with mitochondrial disorders, the mitochondria are dysfunctional and as a result, the cells are denied the energy they need. Because the cells of the brain, muscles, heart, nervous system, and eyes demand the most energy, they are often the most significantly affected areas of the body in someone with a mitochondrial disorder. Possible symptoms may include muscle weakness, hearing impairment, intellectual disabilities, learning disabilities, visual impairment, respiratory disorders, and seizures. Because there is no cure for mitochondrial disorders, treatment focuses on alleviating symptoms and improving quality of life.

FACT

Every year, 1,000 to 4,000 children are born with mitochondrial disease in the United States. When an adult is diagnosed with mitochondrial disease, it is called adult-onset mitochondrial disease. In some cases, late diagnoses are a result of an earlier misdiagnosis. Symptoms may also begin after a severe illness triggers a genetic mutation that was already present.

Proper nutrition is often the primary therapy for mitochondrial disorders, and because seizures are a common symptom, the ketogenic diet is often part of the treatment plan. There have been several studies that show that the ketogenic diet not only helps reduce seizures in those with mitochondrial disorders but also improves symptoms and overall quality of life.

Amyotrophic Lateral Sclerosis (Lou Gehrig's Disease)

Amyotrophic lateral sclerosis, or ALS, became well known when baseball great Lou Gehrig was diagnosed with the extremely rare degenerative disease in 1939. After the diagnosis, the condition became commonly known as Lou Gehrig's disease.

ALS is a progressive neurodegenerative disorder that attacks the nerve cells in the brain and the spinal cord. The disease specifically affects the motor neurons, which control voluntary muscle movement. As the motor neurons die, they are no longer able to send nerve signals to the muscle fibers. When that happens, it can cause muscle weakness, slurred speech, and difficulty swallowing and breathing. Eventually, the muscles begin to atrophy, or become smaller, and the person affected becomes weaker and weaker.

The exact cause of ALS is unknown, but researchers believe that disruptions in the mitochondria in the brain play a role and that changing the type and amount of energy produced in the mitochondria through changes in diet may help those with ALS.

Although there is no cure for the disease, preliminary animal studies have shown that mice that were fed a ketogenic diet experienced a greater reduction in symptoms than mice who weren't. Because these studies were done on mice and not humans, there is no way to say whether humans would benefit the same way, but preliminary results are encouraging.

These conditions are serious and the decision to begin a medical ketogenic diet should not be taken lightly. If you or your child is affected by one of these disorders, consider talking with your physician or a trained nutrition professional about starting a ketogenic diet. If you do decide to implement a medical ketogenic diet, make sure you're closely following the instructions of your healthcare professional to avoid any complications or nutritional deficiencies. You should never start a medical ketogenic diet on your own.

CHAPTER 5

Risks and Concerns

When you mention the term "ketogenic diet" to someone, you'll usually get one of two responses. The first will be something along the lines of, "Oh, I've heard of that. Tell me more." The second will be more like, "Oh, I've heard of that. It might be really dangerous. Be careful." While there are some individuals who should not follow a ketogenic diet, many others can significantly benefit from one. Confusion over the words "ketosis" and "ketoacidosis" is one of the major reasons people are quick to say that a ketogenic diet is dangerous.

Ketosis versus Ketoacidosis

When discussing a ketogenic diet, it's important to differentiate between the terms "ketosis" and "ketoacidosis." A properly planned ketogenic diet is perfectly safe, while ketoacidosis is a dangerous metabolic state that mostly affects type 1 diabetics or those with impaired insulin production.

ESSENTIAL

The levels of ketones associated with ketoacidosis are about three to five times higher than the levels associated with nutritional ketosis. As long as your ketone levels stay in a nutritional ketosis range, you're not at risk for ketoacidosis.

The Basics of Type 1 Diabetes

Insulin is a hormone that allows glucose to enter your cells so that you can obtain energy from the sugar. Type 1 diabetes is a chronic autoimmune condition in which the pancreas produces too little insulin or stops producing insulin completely. Without insulin, glucose cannot enter the cells, so the sugar remains in the bloodstream, accumulating to abnormal levels, and the cells start to starve. A person with type 1 diabetes needs to take insulin, usually through injections or orally, to allow glucose to enter into the cells.

What Is Ketoacidosis?

Ketosis is regulated by insulin. Insulin controls the creation of ketone bodies and regulates the flow of fatty acids into the blood. In a healthy individual, ketosis is tightly controlled; insulin does not allow ketone bodies to reach toxic levels. Because type 1 diabetics do not produce adequate amounts of insulin, their bodies are unable to regulate ketones in the same way. As a result, ketones can accumulate in the blood, turning it into an acidic and potentially dangerous environment. When this happens, it can lead to ketoacidosis, a dangerous metabolic state in which excessive amounts of ketones are produced.

Identifying Ketoacidosis

The signs of ketoacidosis generally appear within 24 hours of the accumulation of toxic ketone levels. Symptoms may include excessive thirst, increased urination, nausea, vomiting, abdominal pain, shortness of breath, weakness, fatigue, and confusion. The presence of ketones will make the breath smell fruity or ammonia-like (although this alone isn't a sign of ketoacidosis—those in nutritional ketosis may also experience fruity-smelling breath). Ketoacidosis is also characterized by a high level of ketones in the urine and high blood sugar.

ALERT

Ketoacidosis is a medical emergency. If left untreated, it can lead to loss of consciousness, coma, and even death. If you experience any of the signs and symptoms of ketoacidosis, seek medical attention immediately.

Purported Risks

In addition to the confusion between ketosis and ketoacidosis, opponents to the ketogenic diet have several other concerns about its safety. Many of these concerns arise from confusion about what the ketogenic diet actually is. Others are common myths that have been circulating for decades, yet are not backed by scientific literature.

Lack of Nutrients

One of the biggest concerns about the ketogenic diet is whether you'll be getting enough nutrients to keep you healthy. Opponents argue that you need a large amount of carbohydrates in your diet to stay healthy and that removing them prevents you from getting all the nutrients you need, but the benefits of carbohydrates, especially grains, are actually overstated.

It is true that your brain needs glucose to function, but your liver can make all of the glucose your brain needs from glycogen stored in the liver. If necessary, your body can also obtain glucose from the protein you eat.

A properly planned ketogenic diet supplies all of the nutrients your body needs to stay healthy and to run efficiently. A particular nutrient of concern is vitamin C, since the richest sources of vitamin C are not permitted on a ketogenic diet; however, a properly planned ketogenic diet, which includes high-quality meat and lots of green vegetables, supplies all of the vitamin C you need.

Heart Disease

On the other end of the spectrum, opponents of the ketogenic diet are also concerned that the diet is just too high in certain nutrients—fat and cholesterol, specifically. The belief is that eating too much fat will eventually lead to high cholesterol in the blood and result in heart troubles such as heart attack and heart disease. As previously mentioned, however, there is a great deal of confusion regarding what causes heart disease and whether fat plays as big a role as many believe it does. The quick answer to this is that scientific evidence does not support the theory that increased dietary fat intake leads to high blood cholesterol levels and heart disease.

This may come as a big surprise, especially if you've been told the opposite all your life, but to understand this concept, you need to understand cholesterol. Cholesterol is not a bad thing. In fact, it's necessary for survival. Cholesterol acts as a precursor to important hormones, including estrogen and testosterone. Your body uses cholesterol to make vitamin D, which plays a role in immune and neuromuscular function, moderates cell growth, and helps maintain calcium levels. Cholesterol also makes up the outer coating of each one of your cells. Without cholesterol, you couldn't live.

On average, the human body contains about 1,000 milligrams of cholesterol at any given time. Most of this cholesterol, about 75 percent, is actually made in the body by your liver. The rest, or 25 percent, comes from the food you eat. Because your body likes to keep cholesterol within a certain range, and does a really good job of regulating it, the amount of cholesterol your liver produces varies based on how much cholesterol you eat. When you eat a lot of dietary cholesterol, the amount of cholesterol your body makes decreases. When the amount of cholesterol in your diet drops, your liver amps up production.

FACT

Your body is not able to absorb all of the cholesterol you eat. In fact, a large percentage of dietary cholesterol never even makes it into your bloodstream; instead, your body excretes it as waste.

So what about saturated fat? Although it's likely you've heard that saturated fat increases cholesterol levels, and thus your risk of heart disease, most long-term studies have shown that this is not the case. In fact, one study published in the journal *Obesity Reviews* in 2012 reported that a diet that is high in saturated fat (and low in carbohydrates) actually lowers the risk of developing heart disease by decreasing triglyceride levels, improving blood pressure, decreasing body mass index, and increasing HDL, or good cholesterol.

Kidney Problems

Because the ketogenic diet is low in carbohydrates, many assume that it's a high-protein diet (as previously mentioned, it's actually a high-fat, moderate-protein diet), and there's a common misconception that eating too much protein can damage the kidneys. While it's true that those with damaged kidneys cannot handle protein as well as those with healthy kidneys, a high-protein diet will not damage the kidneys in otherwise healthy individuals.

There is the potential for kidney stones when following a ketogenic diet. In most cases, kidney stones develop as a result of dehydration. To reduce the risk of developing kidney stones, always make sure you're drinking enough water—at least half your body weight in ounces. If you have kidney trouble, talk with your doctor before starting a ketogenic diet, as it may not be right for you.

When the Ketogenic Diet Should Not Be Used

While the ketogenic diet is safe for most individuals, there are some people who should not follow the diet plan. If you have certain metabolic conditions or health conditions, talk to your doctor before starting a ketogenic diet.

Contraindicated health conditions include:

- Gallbladder disease
- Impaired fat digestion
- History of pancreatitis
- Kidney disease
- Impaired liver function
- Poor nutritional status
- Previous gastric bypass surgery
- Type 1 diabetes
- Impaired insulin production
- Excessive alcohol use
- Carnitine deficiency
- Porphyria

ALERT

For people with metabolic disorders, ketogenic diets pose more risk than benefit and can cause a great deal of harm. If you have one of these conditions, or if you drink alcohol excessively, a ketogenic diet is not for you.

On the other hand, there are other groups of people for whom the ketogenic diet doesn't pose any serious health risks, but it may not necessarily benefit them, either.

Pregnancy

If you're pregnant or trying to become pregnant, a ketogenic diet may not be right for you. A woman is the most fertile when her body feels satisfied and well nourished. Because ketosis is essentially a starvation state, it's a gamble for women trying to become pregnant to try this diet. A high level of ketones in the blood may also pose a risk to a developing fetus. While traditional low-carbohydrate diets are okay during pregnancy, you should not limit your carbohydrates to the point of ketosis if you're pregnant.

High-Intensity Metabolic Conditioning

There are some conflicting views on whether following a ketogenic diet during periods of intense exercise is beneficial or not. Some athletes claim that ketosis boosts energy, while others, usually those who do high-intensity exercises such as sprints or CrossFit workouts, become burned out faster.

High-intensity exercises require glucose, and although your body can make glucose from protein and fat, it's doesn't do it at the rate at which you need it to sustain high-intensity workouts. Because of this, your body may turn to stored muscle glycogen, which depletes fairly quickly, and your performance may decrease. When you're burned out and your glycogen stores are depleted, you're more likely to have compromised form and sustain an injury during a workout.

Testing Your Ketone Levels

Once you've entered a state of ketosis, the goal is to stay there. The longer you remain in ketosis, the better your body gets at burning ketones for fuel and the better you'll feel. Testing your ketones will also allow you to monitor your ketone levels so that you'll know if they're getting too high. You can determine whether you're in ketosis, and monitor your ketone levels, using several different at-home test options.

Urine Test

Most drugstores carry urine strips that measure the amount of ketones in your urine. These urine strips test the pH of your urine and can give you a general idea of the level of ketones; however, they have their limitations.

There are three major types of ketones present in the blood when you've reached a state of ketosis: acetoacetate (AcAc), beta-hydroxybutyrate or (BHB), and acetone, which is a byproduct of acetoacetate. After a few weeks on the ketogenic diet, levels of ketones begin to rise and your body starts to use them as fuel. Once you become keto-adapted, which takes another few weeks, the muscles convert AcAc ketones into BHB ketones. So why does this matter? The urine ketone test strips only measure for AcAc ketones, so while they're great for measuring your ketone levels when you're new to a ketogenic diet, they might not give you an accurate picture as your body becomes adapted to using ketones as fuel.

Also, as you become keto-adapted and your body begins to efficiently use ketones as fuel, you'll excrete fewer ketones in your urine. This means that a urine ketone test may show no ketones at all even though you're actually in the optimal state of ketosis. Changes in hydration status also affect the amount of ketones in your urine. A high water intake will lower the concentration of ketones in the urine. Because it's important to stay well hydrated on a ketogenic diet, you may see numbers that don't give you an accurate picture.

Blood Test

Because urine testing is not as accurate over the long term, many people who are serious about staying in ketosis have turned to blood meters to test ketones. To test your blood ketone levels, you'll prick your finger with a lancet, which is included in the blood meter kit, and then place a drop of blood on a specialized testing strip. The testing strip goes into the blood meter and gives you a reading on the screen.

Interpreting the Numbers

It's best to measure your blood ketone levels in the morning on an empty stomach since certain things—for instance, a high-fat meal—can affect the reading. A blood ketone level of below 0.5 mmol/L (millimoles per liter) is not considered ketosis. Once you reach a blood ketone level of 0.5 mmol/L to 1.5 mmol/L, you've entered a state of light nutritional ketosis. Here it's likely that you'll experience some weight loss, but the effects won't be optimal. Optimal ketosis is defined as having a blood ketone level of 1.5 mmol/L to 3.0 mmol/L. This is the state recommended for maximum fat burning. Ketone levels higher than 3.0 mmol/L are not necessary, and this is where ketosis has the potential to become dangerous. There is also anecdotal evidence that having a ketone level higher than the optimal range may actually inhibit fat loss.

When to Test

When you test your ketone levels is at least as important as the method you use to test. Because ketone levels fluctuate throughout the day and after meals, you have to be strategic about when you test to get an accurate reading. High-fat meals, especially those that contain a lot of medium-chain triglycerides, will have a direct effect on ketone levels, so avoid testing immediately after meals. Intense aerobic exercise will also increase ketone levels. As a general rule, ketone levels tend to be lower in the morning than in the evening because of all the fat you eat during the day. Testing in the morning right when you wake up may give you the most accurate results.

ESSENTIAL

For the most accurate long-term results, it's a good idea to test your ketone levels around the same time every day. If you have trouble remembering, set an alarm on your cell phone or write yourself a note by your bedside to test your levels right when you wake up.

Staying Safe and Achieving Success

Once you and your healthcare provider have decided that a ketogenic diet is right for you, there are a number of things you can do to ensure that you not only achieve your goals but also stay safe on the diet plan.

Eat Enough

A ketogenic diet is not about excessively restricting calories. Although you do have to stay within a certain caloric range depending on your individual characteristics, you always want to make sure you're eating enough. Restricting carbohydrates and calories too much can leave you feeling tired and moody and can hinder your weight-loss progress.

A ketogenic diet isn't about starving yourself; it's about providing yourself with all of the calories and nutrients you need while restricting carbohydrate intake. As you lose weight, you may have to adjust the amount of calories you need, so make sure to monitor your progress and re-evaluate your diet plan whenever necessary.

Vary Your Food Choices

As with any other diet plan, varying your food choices as much as possible will help ensure that you're getting all of the nutrients you need to stay healthy. If you eat the same thing over and over, day after day, you may not be getting a certain vitamin or mineral that you need. A ketogenic diet is more restrictive than other diet plans, but that doesn't mean you don't have options. Familiarize yourself with your options and vary your plate as much as possible.

Consider Supplements

Many people can get all of the nutrients they need through a balanced ketogenic diet. However, some individuals may need supplementation with specific nutrients. This largely depends on individual characteristics. If you feel that you're doing everything right, but you still don't feel great on a ketogenic diet, contact a functional medicine practitioner or a functional nutritionist. These healthcare practitioners will be able to do the appropriate testing to determine if you have any nutritional deficiencies or identify any areas where your diet may be lacking. Based on this information, a functional medicine practitioner will be able to recommend specific supplements for you.

There are certain supplements that tend to be the most popular for people following a ketogenic diet. Leucine and lysine are two amino acids that help support ketosis and allow you a little more wiggle room with your protein intake. Although vitamin D levels tend to be low in the American population as a whole, those who follow a ketogenic diet may be at a higher risk of becoming deficient. Taking coconut oil as a supplement, 1 to 2 tablespoons per day, can help you reach your fat goals and help prevent constipation while on the diet.

Troubleshooting Constipation

Constipation is a common concern for those on a ketogenic diet, especially those who are in the early stages. If you're experiencing constipation on a ketogenic diet, there are some steps you can take to get things moving again.

ALERT

Bowel movements are extremely important because they allow the body to eliminate waste and prevent toxins from accumulating in the body. You should be having a bowel movement at least once a day, although once after every meal is ideal.

In addition to taking 1 to 2 tablespoons of coconut oil each day, drink adequate amounts of water (half of your body weight in ounces). If you're 200 pounds, this means 100 ounces of water every day. You also need to make sure you're getting enough salt, which helps maintain water balance and replenish sodium levels. Constipation may also be a sign that your protein intake is too high and your fat intake isn't high enough.

Achieving success on a ketogenic diet may take some trial and error and a little bit of practice, but once you get into the routine and reach a state of optimal ketosis, your body will adjust accordingly. If you experience any uncomfortable symptoms or hit any roadblocks, contact a functional medicine doctor or a functional nutritionist who can help you troubleshoot and overcome any hurdles.

CHAPTER 6

Breakfast

Sausage Quiche

This quiche holds up well in the fridge, so it's a good choice when meal planning. You can prepare the quiche on Sunday, put each serving in a plastic container in the fridge, and eat it for breakfast all week.

INGREDIENTS | SERVES 12

12 large eggs
¼ cup heavy cream
½ teaspoon salt
¼ teaspoon black pepper
12 ounces sugar-free breakfast sausage
2 cups shredded Cheddar cheese

Double-Check Your Sausage

A lot of commercially prepared sausages contain corn syrup, which not only is unhealthy but ups the carbohydrate count of your meal. If you can't find breakfast sausage that doesn't contain added sugar, replace the sausage in this recipe with ground pork seasoned with salt, pepper, garlic powder, and sage.

1. Preheat oven to 375°F.

2. Whisk eggs, heavy cream, salt, and pepper together in a large bowl.

3. Add breakfast sausage and Cheddar cheese.

4. Pour mixture into a greased 9" × 13" casserole dish.

5. Bake for 25 minutes. Cut into 12 squares and serve.

Bacon-Wrapped Egg Cups

To give this recipe a little kick, replace the Cheddar cheese with pepper jack and add a pinch of red pepper flakes to the eggs while you're whisking.

INGREDIENTS | SERVES 12

12 slices sugar-free bacon
12 large eggs
½ cup heavy cream
½ teaspoon salt
¼ teaspoon black pepper
½ cup shredded Cheddar cheese
2 cups chopped and steamed broccoli

Be Choosy with Bacon

Like commercially prepared sausage, bacon often contains added sugar in the form of maple syrup or brown sugar. Look for uncured varieties at the supermarket or ask your local butcher to track down some sugar-free bacon for you.

1. Preheat oven to 350°F.

2. Grease each well of a 12-cup muffin tin with butter or coconut oil.

3. Cook bacon in a medium skillet over medium heat until almost crisp. When bacon is fully cooked, quickly line each well of the muffin tin with a piece of bacon.

4. Whisk eggs, heavy cream, salt, and pepper together in a large mixing bowl. Add cheese and chopped broccoli and stir.

5. Pour an equal amount of mixture into each well of the muffin tin.

6. Bake for 20 minutes or until lightly browned on top and firm throughout.

7. Allow to cool for 10 minutes and then remove egg cups from muffin tins. Store in refrigerator.

Western Scrambled Eggs

You can increase the fat content of this recipe by adding chopped avocado to the scrambled eggs once you remove them from the heat.

INGREDIENTS | SERVES 4

8 large eggs

¼ cup heavy cream

1 teaspoon salt

½ teaspoon black pepper

1 tablespoon butter

½ cup diced sugar-free ham

½ cup chopped onion

½ cup chopped red and green peppers

1 cup shredded Cheddar cheese

Chopped scallions for garnish (optional)

1. Whisk eggs, cream, salt, and black pepper together in a large mixing bowl.

2. Melt butter in a medium skillet over medium heat. Add egg mixture and stir. When eggs start to scramble, add ham, onion, and peppers. Continue to stir until eggs are almost cooked. Add cheese and stir until cooked.

3. Garnish with scallions, if desired.

Almond Butter Muffins

For some variation, replace the almond butter in this recipe with another one of your favorite nut butters. Cashew butter, peanut butter, and sunflower seed butter work well.

INGREDIENTS | SERVES 12

⅔ cup almond flour
¼ cup granulated erythritol
1 teaspoon ground cinnamon
¼ cup unsweetened almond butter
2 tablespoons butter
1 tablespoon coconut oil
1 teaspoon vanilla extract
4 large eggs
¼ cup heavy cream

Learning about Erythritol

Erythritol is a naturally derived sugar substitute that looks and tastes like sugar but has almost no calories and a low glycemic load, which means it doesn't significantly affect your blood sugar levels. Erythritol comes in two forms, granulated and powdered, and can be used in place of sugar in any recipe, although it is only 70 percent as sweet.

1. Preheat oven to 350°F.

2. Mix together almond flour, erythritol, and cinnamon in a medium mixing bowl.

3. In a separate bowl, beat almond butter, butter, coconut oil, vanilla extract, eggs, and heavy cream together until smooth.

4. Add almond flour mixture to almond butter mixture and stir until smooth.

5. Put a paper cupcake liner in each well of a 12-cup muffin tin. Fill each paper cup with batter.

6. Bake for 20 minutes or until a toothpick inserted in the center comes out clean.

7. Remove from muffin tin and allow to cool before serving.

Eggs Benedict

Traditional Eggs Benedict calls for Canadian bacon, but you can use sugar-free bacon, sugar-free sausage, or prosciutto in place of the Canadian bacon.

INGREDIENTS | SERVES 2

1 tablespoon butter

4 large eggs

4 slices sugar-free Canadian bacon

½ large avocado, cut into 4 slices

1 cup Hollandaise Sauce (see recipe in Chapter 9)

1. Heat up a medium skillet over medium-high heat and add the butter. Crack eggs into pan. Cook for 2 minutes and then flip eggs, using care not to break yolks. Cook for another 2 minutes or until white is completely cooked, but yolk is still runny. Transfer eggs to a plate.

2. Top each egg with a slice of Canadian bacon and a slice of avocado. Pour ¼ cup of the sauce mixture onto each egg.

Bacon Hash

Turn this into a complete meal by adding a couple of poached or over-easy eggs on top. You can also mix this bacon hash into some scrambled eggs.

INGREDIENTS | SERVES 4

6 slices sugar-free bacon
2 cups chopped cauliflower
1 medium onion, diced
2 cloves garlic, minced
½ teaspoon salt
½ teaspoon black pepper
½ teaspoon garlic powder

1. Cook bacon in a medium skillet over medium heat until crispy, about 10 minutes. Remove from pan and let cool, then dice.

2. Add chopped cauliflower, diced onion, and minced garlic to the skillet. Cook 5 minutes over medium heat, or until cauliflower starts to brown. Add salt, black pepper, garlic powder, and diced bacon. Stir until combined.

3. Remove from heat and serve.

Ham, Cheese, and Egg Casserole

Mozzarella and Cheddar cheese give this dish a mild cheesy flavor, but you can use any type of shredded cheese you want.

INGREDIENTS | SERVES 6

4 cups broccoli florets
12 large eggs
2 cups cooked diced sugar-free ham
½ cup shredded mozzarella cheese
½ cup shredded Cheddar cheese
¼ cup chopped scallions

Bunches of Broccoli

One cup of chopped broccoli contains only 6 grams of carbohydrates, half of which come from fiber. In addition to being low in carbohydrates, broccoli is high in vitamin C, a nutrient that you definitely need when following a ketogenic diet.

1. Preheat oven to 375°F.

2. Fill a large pot with water and bring to a boil. Blanch broccoli by putting in boiling water for 2–3 minutes.

3. Put eggs, ham, mozzarella, Cheddar, and scallions in a large bowl and whisk until combined. Add broccoli.

4. Pour into a 9" × 13" baking dish and cook for 35 minutes or until eggs are cooked through.

Scrambled Eggs with Bacon

This is a simple recipe, but it's a staple for a ketogenic diet. Scrambled eggs and bacon are typically thought of as breakfast food, but you can eat this whenever you need a quick dose of protein and fat.

INGREDIENTS | SERVES 2

4 slices sugar-free bacon
6 large eggs
¼ cup heavy cream
¼ teaspoon salt
¼ teaspoon black pepper

1. Cook bacon in a medium skillet over medium heat until crispy, about 10 minutes. Remove bacon from pan and dice.

2. Crack eggs into a medium bowl and whisk together with heavy cream, salt, and pepper. Add egg mixture to bacon grease in pan and stir until scrambled. Add diced bacon to eggs and stir.

3. Remove from heat and serve immediately.

Spicy Sausage Egg Cups

If you don't like spice, omit or use less of the red pepper flakes. You could also substitute with garlic powder.

INGREDIENTS | SERVES 6

½ pound ground pork
½ teaspoon dried sage
½ teaspoon salt
½ teaspoon black pepper
¼ teaspoon red pepper flakes
¼ medium yellow onion, chopped
¼ cup chopped zucchini
12 large eggs
1 large avocado, diced

Versatile Zucchini

Zucchini is a good source of vitamin C and vitamin B_6, and at only 2.5 net grams of carbohydrates per cup, it makes a great addition to any ketogenic meal. Because zucchini is extremely mild tasting, you can add it to any meal without significantly changing the flavor.

1. Preheat oven to 350°F.

2. Heat a large skillet over medium heat and add ground pork, sage, salt, black pepper, and red pepper. Cook until meat is no longer pink. Remove pork with a slotted spoon and set aside. Add onion and zucchini to pan and sauté until tender, about 4 minutes. Add cooked onion and zucchini to pork mixture in a medium bowl.

3. Add eggs to pork mixture and stir until combined. Oil each well of a 12-cup muffin tin with a small amount of coconut oil and pour mixture evenly into each well.

4. Bake for 30 minutes or until egg is cooked through.

5. Top each egg cup with a few pieces of avocado.

Spinach and Mozzarella Egg Bake

Use only the green stalks of the scallions for this recipe, but don't throw the white parts out! Save them to use in other recipes.

INGREDIENTS | SERVES 4

1 tablespoon olive oil
4 cups baby spinach
¾ cup shredded mozzarella cheese
¾ cup shredded Colby jack cheese
¼ cup chopped scallions
8 large eggs
½ teaspoon salt
½ teaspoon black pepper

1. Preheat oven to 375°F.

2. Heat olive oil in a medium skillet over medium heat and add spinach. Sauté until wilted. Transfer spinach to a 9" × 9" baking dish.

3. Put remaining ingredients in a medium bowl and whisk until combined. Pour egg mixture on top of spinach.

4. Bake for 30 minutes or until eggs are no longer runny. Serve warm.

Bacon-and-Egg-Stuffed Avocados

Take these stuffed avocados out of the oven as soon as the egg is cooked through. If you cook an avocado too long, it develops a bitter, unpleasant taste.

INGREDIENTS | SERVES 2

2 large avocados

4 strips cooked sugar-free bacon, crumbled

4 large eggs

¼ teaspoon sea salt

¼ teaspoon black pepper

A for Avocado

Avocados are the ketogenic dieter's dream. A single avocado contains almost 30 grams of fat and only 3 grams of net carbohydrates. You can easily increase the fat content of any meal by adding a few slices of avocado.

1. Preheat oven to 400°F.

2. Cut avocados in half lengthwise and remove the pit. Scoop some avocado out of each half to create a well.

3. Sprinkle 1 strip crumbled bacon into each avocado well. Crack 1 egg directly into each avocado half. Season with salt and black pepper. Place avocados on a baking sheet.

4. Bake for 15 minutes or until egg is cooked to desired doneness.

CHAPTER 7

Lunch

Tuna and Egg Salad

This tuna and egg salad keeps well in the refrigerator for a week. Save time during the week by doubling or tripling the recipe and having it for lunch all week.

INGREDIENTS | SERVES 2

2 large hard-boiled eggs

2 (6-ounce) cans tuna

¼ cup Homemade Mayonnaise (see recipe in Chapter 9)

¼ cup diced white onion

¼ cup sugar-free relish

¼ teaspoon salt

¼ teaspoon black pepper

Put eggs in a medium mixing bowl and mash with a fork. Add tuna and mayonnaise and mash together until ingredients are combined. Stir in onion, relish, salt, and pepper.

Oil or Water?

Tuna comes packed in oil or water. You can up the fat content of this meal by choosing the tuna that's packed in oil.

"Mac" 'n' Cheese

You can make this "Mac" 'n' Cheese into a vegetarian option by simply omitting the crushed pork rinds.

INGREDIENTS | SERVES 6

6 cups cauliflower florets
3 ounces cream cheese
1 cup heavy cream
1½ cups shredded Cheddar cheese, divided
½ teaspoon black pepper
¼ teaspoon garlic powder
¼ teaspoon salt
½ cup crushed pork rinds

1. Preheat oven to 375°F.

2. Fill a double boiler with water and bring water to a boil. Cut cauliflower into small pieces and place in the top portion of the double boiler. Steam until tender, about 5 minutes.

3. Remove cauliflower from double boiler and place in a strainer.

4. Melt cream cheese in a medium saucepan over medium heat. Add heavy cream and whisk until combined. Whisk in 1 cup of Cheddar cheese, pepper, garlic powder, and salt. Once cheese has melted, remove from heat.

5. Transfer strained cauliflower to a 9" × 9" baking dish. Pour in cheese mixture and toss to coat cauliflower. Sprinkle remaining ½ cup of cheese and pork rinds on top. Bake until bubbly, about 20 minutes.

Chicken and Avocado Salad

Precooked canned chicken makes this recipe a cinch to whip up, but if you have extra time, you can cook some boneless, skinless chicken breasts, shred them, and use that instead.

INGREDIENTS | SERVES 2

1 (12.5-ounce) can shredded chicken breast

1 medium avocado, cubed

¼ cup Homemade Mayonnaise (see recipe in Chapter 9)

2 tablespoons sliced black olives

¼ teaspoon garlic salt

¼ teaspoon black pepper

⅛ teaspoon paprika

1 teaspoon fresh lemon juice

1 teaspoon olive oil

Put all ingredients in a medium mixing bowl and mash with a fork until combined.

Deli Roll-Ups

Instead of purchasing prepared chive cream cheese, you can make your own by combining plain cream cheese with minced onions and dried chives.

INGREDIENTS | SERVES 2

8 ounces sugar-free deli ham, sliced
½ cup chive cream cheese
1 cup chopped baby spinach
1 red bell pepper, sliced

Pick Your Bell

Red peppers contain more carbohydrates than green peppers. If you need to reduce the carbohydrate content for this recipe, you can swap out the red pepper for a green one.

1. Lay out each slice of ham flat. Take 1 tablespoon of cream cheese and spread it on a slice of ham. Repeat for the remaining slices.

2. Put 2 tablespoons of chopped spinach on top of the cream cheese on each slice.

3. Divide bell pepper into 8 equal portions and put each portion on top of spinach.

4. Roll up the ham and secure with a toothpick. Eat immediately or refrigerate until ready to serve.

Ham and Cheese Casserole

Allow the cream cheese to reach room temperature before starting this recipe. Softened cream cheese is much easier to work with than cream cheese fresh from the fridge.

INGREDIENTS | SERVES 6

6 cups cauliflower florets

½ cup cream cheese, softened

½ cup heavy cream

¼ cup coconut cream

2½ cups cooked cubed sugar-free ham

1 cup shredded Cheddar cheese

1½ tablespoons grated Parmesan cheese

¼ cup chopped scallions

½ teaspoon salt

¼ teaspoon black pepper

Corralling Coconut Cream

Coconut cream is the solid portion of the coconut milk you buy in a can. You can easily separate the cream from the milk by refrigerating a can of full-fat milk for a few hours. When it's chilled, open the can and scoop out the solid part on top—this is the coconut cream and the part that contains most of the fat. Save the milk that's left at the bottom for a smoothie or use it in another recipe.

1. Preheat oven to 350°F. Bring a large pot of water to a boil and add cauliflower. Boil until cauliflower is fork tender, about 5–10 minutes. Strain cauliflower and return to pot.

2. Put cream cheese, heavy cream, and coconut cream in a medium mixing bowl and beat with a handheld beater until smooth. Transfer cream cheese mixture to cauliflower pot and stir until cauliflower is coated. Add in ham, Cheddar cheese, Parmesan cheese, scallions, salt, and pepper and stir until combined.

3. Transfer mixture to a 9" × 9" baking dish and bake until cheese is melted and casserole is bubbly, about 30 minutes. Serve hot.

Stuffed Avocados

Choose avocados that are ripe but still firm for this recipe—dark and slightly soft, but not mushy.

INGREDIENTS | SERVES 2

1 large avocado

1 (6-ounce) can tuna

2 tablespoons Homemade Mayonnaise (see recipe in Chapter 9)

½ medium green bell pepper, chopped

¼ teaspoon dried minced onion

⅛ teaspoon garlic salt

⅛ teaspoon black pepper

1. Cut avocado in half lengthwise and remove the pit. Set aside.

2. Put tuna, mayonnaise, bell pepper, dried onion, garlic salt, and black pepper in a medium mixing bowl and mash together with a fork until combined.

3. Scoop half of the mixture into each half of the avocado.

Meatball "Sub"

*For another variation of this recipe, use sliced mozzarella cheese
in place of provolone and ½ pound of lamb instead of pork.*

INGREDIENTS | SERVES 6 (18 MEATBALLS)

1 pound ground beef
½ pound ground pork
2 tablespoons grated Parmesan cheese
2 large eggs
¼ cup chopped fresh basil
2 tablespoons minced fresh parsley
1 tablespoon minced garlic
1 teaspoon salt
½ teaspoon black pepper
6 slices provolone cheese
1 cup Marinara Sauce (see recipe in Chapter 9)

1. Preheat oven to 325°F.

2. Mix beef, pork, Parmesan cheese, eggs, basil, parsley, garlic, salt, and pepper in a large mixing bowl until well combined.

3. Roll meat mixture into 1" balls and place about 1" apart on a baking sheet. Bake until cooked through, about 15 minutes. Remove meatballs from the oven and set aside to cool for a few minutes.

4. Place 1 slice of provolone cheese flat on a plate and put 3 meatballs on one side of it. Pour ⅙ of the marinara sauce over the meatballs. Fold the other side of the cheese over the meatballs.

Roast Beef Lettuce Wraps

These lettuce wraps are incredibly easy to take with you on the go. When you're in a rush or have a busy day, prepare a few in the morning and pack them away for lunch later in the day.

INGREDIENTS | SERVES 4

8 large iceberg lettuce leaves

8 ounces (8 slices) rare roast beef

¼ cup Homemade Mayonnaise (see recipe in Chapter 9)

8 slices provolone cheese

1 cup baby spinach

Iceberg Lettuce

The iceberg lettuce in this recipe serves mainly as a vehicle for the meat, since it contains very few nutrients, aside from being high in water. You can use romaine lettuce in place of iceberg, but iceberg tends to hold its shape better.

1. Wash lettuce leaves and pat them dry, being careful not to rip them.

2. Place 1 slice of roast beef in each lettuce wrap.

3. Spread ½ tablespoon of mayonnaise on each piece of roast beef.

4. Top mayonnaise with 1 slice of provolone cheese and ⅛ cup of baby spinach.

5. Roll lettuce up around toppings. Serve immediately.

Spicy Chicken and Avocado Casserole

*You can replace the chicken in this recipe with canned tuna,
ground beef or pork, or diced chunks of ham.*

INGREDIENTS | SERVES 6

2 large avocados, roughly chopped

2 tablespoons coconut oil

1 small onion, diced

1 medium green bell pepper, diced

3 (12.5-ounce) cans shredded chicken breast

½ cup sour cream

½ cup Homemade Mayonnaise (see recipe in Chapter 9)

1½ cups shredded Cheddar cheese, divided

⅛ teaspoon red pepper flakes

¼ teaspoon salt

¼ teaspoon black pepper

Go Crazy for Coconut Oil

Coconut oil is a staple in the ketogenic diet. The oil is resistant to high heat, so unlike olive oil, it doesn't oxidize with high temperatures. Coconut oil also contains medium-chain triglycerides, a type of fat that can help boost metabolism.

1. Preheat oven to 350°F.

2. Spread chopped avocados along the bottom of a 9" × 13" baking pan.

3. Heat coconut oil in a medium skillet over medium-high heat. Add diced onions and cook until lightly browned, about 3 minutes. Add bell pepper to pan and cook until soft, another 3 minutes. Remove from heat.

4. Place chicken, sour cream, mayonnaise, 1 cup of Cheddar cheese, red pepper, salt, and black pepper in a medium mixing bowl and stir until combined. Add onions and bell peppers.

5. Spoon mixture over avocados. Top with remaining ½ cup of Cheddar cheese.

6. Bake for 20 minutes, or until cheese is slightly browned and casserole is bubbling.

7. Allow to cool slightly before serving.

Fried Chicken

If you want extra-crispy fried chicken, dip the chicken breasts in pork rind mixture, then egg mixture, then pork rind mixture again. This will create a thick coating and really crisp it up.

INGREDIENTS | SERVES 4

¾ cup crushed pork rinds

¼ cup grated Parmesan cheese

½ teaspoon garlic powder

½ teaspoon onion powder

½ teaspoon dried minced onion

¼ teaspoon salt

½ teaspoon black pepper

2 large eggs

1 pound or 4 (4-ounce) boneless, skinless chicken breasts

2 tablespoons coconut oil

Picking Pork Rinds

All pork rinds are not created equal. When choosing pork rinds, read the ingredient list and choose one that contains only pork skin and pork fat or pork skin and salt. You want to avoid pork rinds that are cooked in processed lard.

1. Put pork rinds, Parmesan cheese, garlic powder, onion powder, minced onion, salt, and black pepper in a large mixing bowl and stir until well mixed.

2. Crack eggs into a separate bowl and whisk.

3. Dip each chicken breast into eggs and then coat in pork rind mixture, making sure the chicken is completely covered.

4. Heat coconut oil in a skillet over medium-high heat. When coconut oil is hot, place chicken breasts into pan. Let cook for 5–7 minutes or until pork rind crust is browned. Flip chicken over and let cook for another 5–7 minutes until cooked through.

5. Serve hot.

Pepperoni Pizza Casserole

Instead of pepperoni, you can use salami or prosciutto in this recipe. Just read the ingredients and make sure that the cured meats don't contain any added sugar.

INGREDIENTS | SERVES 6

6 cups cauliflower florets (about 1 large cauliflower head)

2 tablespoons butter

¼ cup heavy cream

2 tablespoons grated Parmesan cheese

1 teaspoon Italian seasoning

1 cup mozzarella cheese, divided

½ cup Marinara Sauce (see recipe in Chapter 9)

12 slices sugar-free pepperoni

1. Preheat oven to 375°F. Bring a large pot of water to a boil and add cauliflower florets. Boil until fork tender, about 5–7 minutes.

2. Strain cauliflower and put into a food processor or blender. While cauliflower is still hot, add butter and heavy cream, and process or blend until smooth. Add Parmesan cheese, Italian seasoning, and ¼ cup mozzarella cheese and process until smooth.

3. Pour cauliflower mixture into a 9" × 9" pan and spread it out evenly. Pour marinara sauce over cauliflower mixture.

4. Top with remaining mozzarella cheese and pepperoni. Bake for 20 minutes, or until cheese is slightly browned and casserole is bubbling.

Turkey Avocado Rolls

Lemon pepper has a strong taste, so in this recipe, a little goes a long way. If you don't like the zing of lemon, try garlic pepper in place of the lemon pepper or just omit the spice blend completely.

INGREDIENTS | SERVES 4

12 slices (12 ounces) turkey breast

12 slices Swiss cheese

3 cups baby spinach

1 large avocado, cut into 12 slices

¼ cup Homemade Mayonnaise (see recipe in Chapter 9)

¼ teaspoon lemon pepper

1. Lay out the slices of turkey breast flat and place a slice of Swiss cheese on top of each one.

2. Top each slice with ¼ cup baby spinach and 3 slices of avocado. Drizzle with 1 teaspoon of mayonnaise.

3. Sprinkle each "sandwich" with lemon pepper. Roll up sandwiches and secure with toothpicks. Serve immediately or refrigerate until ready to serve.

Check Your Spices

It may come as a surprise, but many commercial spices contain sugar or hydrogenated fats. Don't assume that an ingredient, such as lemon pepper, is free of carbohydrates until you check the label. If it contains sugar, ditch it and find one that doesn't. When it comes to herbs and spices, there are plenty of sugar-free options out there.

Breadless BLT

When cooking the tomato for this recipe, you just want to char it slightly, not cook it through. If it gets too soft, it won't hold up as well.

INGREDIENTS | SERVES 2

6 slices sugar-free bacon

1 large tomato, cut into 4 equal slices

4 leaves romaine lettuce

½ large avocado, sliced

2 tablespoons Homemade Mayonnaise (see recipe in Chapter 9)

1. Cook bacon in a medium skillet over medium heat until crisp. Remove bacon and return bacon fat to heat.

2. Place each tomato slice in bacon fat and cook for 1 minute. Remove from pan and set aside.

3. Top each of 2 tomato slices with 2 slices of romaine lettuce, ¼ of avocado, and 1 tablespoon mayonnaise.

4. Cover with remaining tomato slices.

Portobello Pizzas

This is a basic pizza combination, but you can use whatever combination of toppings you want. Try sausage and green peppers or prosciutto and mushrooms.

INGREDIENTS | SERVES 4

4 large portobello mushrooms
4 teaspoons olive oil
1 cup Marinara Sauce (see recipe in Chapter 9)
1 cup shredded mozzarella cheese
12 slices sugar-free pepperoni

The Versatile Portobello

Portobello mushrooms are larger, more mature versions of the common white mushroom. The portobello mushroom has a rich, meaty flavor and texture and, because of this, it's often used as a substitute for meat in vegetarian recipes.

1. Preheat oven to 375°F.

2. Remove stems from mushrooms and brush each cap inside and outside with 1 teaspoon olive oil. Place on a foil-lined baking sheet and bake stem side down for 10 minutes.

3. Remove mushrooms from oven and fill each cap with ¼ cup marinara sauce, ¼ cup mozzarella cheese, and 3 slices of pepperoni.

4. Return to oven and cook for another 10 minutes or until cheese is lightly browned and bubbly. Serve hot.

Chicken Cordon Bleu Casserole

Traditional chicken cordon bleu contains ham, chicken, and Swiss cheese, but if you're not a fan of Swiss cheese, swap it out for a cheese with a milder flavor, such as provolone or mozzarella.

INGREDIENTS | SERVES 4

2 cups cooked chopped chicken breast
1 cup cooked diced sugar-free ham
1 cup cubed Swiss cheese
½ cup heavy cream
½ cup sour cream
½ cup cream cheese
½ teaspoon granulated garlic
½ teaspoon granulated onion
¼ teaspoon salt
¼ teaspoon black pepper
½ cup crushed pork rinds

1. Preheat oven to 350°F.

2. Mix cooked chicken and diced ham and spread out in the bottom of a 9" × 13" baking dish.

3. Sprinkle Swiss cheese on top of chicken and ham.

4. Put heavy cream, sour cream, and cheese in a medium saucepan and heat over medium heat until cream cheese is melted and mixture is smooth. Add garlic, onion, salt, and pepper. Pour mixture over chicken, ham, and Swiss cheese.

5. Sprinkle pork rinds across casserole. Bake for 30 minutes, or until slightly browned and cheese is bubbly.

CHAPTER 8

Dinner

Stuffed Chicken Breast

You can use frozen spinach in place of the fresh spinach for this recipe. Just make sure it's completely thawed and drained before use or the filling will be runny.

INGREDIENTS | SERVES 4

1 pound (4 individual) boneless, skinless chicken breasts

¼ cup cream cheese, softened

¼ cup sour cream

1 (10-ounce) package fresh spinach, chopped

⅓ cup chopped fresh basil

1 tablespoon minced green onions

½ cup shredded pepper jack cheese

2 cloves garlic, minced

¼ teaspoon salt

¼ teaspoon black pepper

1. Preheat oven to 375°F.

2. Cut a slit into the side of each chicken breast to create a pocket.

3. Combine all other ingredients in a medium bowl and beat until smooth.

4. Fill each chicken breast with ¼ of the mixture and secure pocket closed with toothpicks.

5. Place chicken breasts in a baking dish and cook for 35 minutes, or until chicken is no longer pink.

Baked Salmon with Garlic Aioli

Watch the clock when marinating this recipe. If you leave raw fish sitting in lemon juice too long, the fish will start to "cook." The citric acid in the lemon juice can change the proteins in the fish, turning the flesh firm and opaque, similar to how it would look and feel if it had been cooked with heat.

INGREDIENTS | SERVES 4

3 cloves garlic, minced
¼ cup extra-virgin olive oil
¼ cup melted butter
1 tablespoon lemon juice
½ teaspoon salt
½ teaspoon black pepper
1 teaspoon dried parsley
1 pound (4 individual) salmon fillets
½ cup Garlic Aioli (see recipe in Chapter 9)

Outstanding Omega-3s

A 4-ounce fillet of salmon contains just about 15 grams of fat. Most of this fat comes in the form of omega-3 fatty acids, which promote brain health and heart health and help protect against cancer and autoimmune diseases such as rheumatoid arthritis and lupus.

1. Combine garlic, olive oil, butter, lemon juice, salt, pepper, and parsley in a mixing bowl. Place salmon in a baking dish and pour marinade on top. Refrigerate for 1 hour.

2. Preheat oven to 350°F.

3. Put salmon in oven and bake for 35 minutes or until fish flakes easily with a fork.

4. Remove from oven and top each piece of salmon with ⅛ cup of garlic aioli.

Taco Bowls

If you prefer to mimic more traditional tacos, you can place the filling for this recipe into large leaves of iceberg lettuce and fold them up like tacos.

INGREDIENTS | SERVES 4

1 pound 85/15 lean ground beef

2 tablespoons taco seasoning

1 large avocado, chopped

1 cup shredded Cheddar cheese

1 cup sour cream

½ cup sliced black olives

Cilantro, chopped (optional)

1. Brown ground beef in a large skillet over medium heat. Without draining fat, add taco seasoning and stir until liquid is absorbed and beef is covered with seasoning.

2. Put ¼ of the beef into each of four bowls. Top beef in each bowl with ¼ avocado, ¼ cup of Cheddar cheese, ¼ cup of sour cream, and ⅛ cup of sliced olives.

3. Garnish with cilantro, if desired.

Choosing Your Meats

Whenever possible, choose high-quality meats such as grass-fed beef and free-range, organic chicken. These animals are allowed to eat food that is a part of their natural diet, rather than being force-fed grains and other foods that they are not biologically designed to eat. Animals that consume their natural diet are better for you nutritionally.

Meatloaf

You don't need bread crumbs to hold meatloaf together. This recipe uses an egg instead, which keeps the carbohydrates low while also increasing fat and protein content.

INGREDIENTS | SERVES 4

2 tablespoons butter

1 large yellow onion

4 cloves garlic, minced

4 slices cooked sugar-free bacon

1 pound 85/15 lean ground beef

1 large egg

1 teaspoon dried thyme

1 teaspoon dried parsley

½ teaspoon dry mustard

½ teaspoon salt

¼ teaspoon black pepper

The Power of Parsley

Parsley isn't just a garnish. The herb is rich in vitamin C and vitamin A, so it helps keep your immune system, bones, and nervous system strong. Parsley also helps flush out excess water from the body and keeps your kidneys healthy.

1. Preheat oven to 350°F.

2. Heat butter in a large skillet over medium-high heat until melted. Add onions and garlic and sauté until softened, 3–4 minutes. Remove from heat and set aside to cool.

3. Chop bacon and put in a large mixing bowl. Add ground beef, egg, herbs, spices, and garlic and onion mixture and mix until evenly incorporated.

4. Transfer meat mixture to a 9" × 5" loaf pan.

5. Cook for 1 hour or until a meat thermometer inserted in the center reads 165°F.

Shrimp Scampi

This dish is easy to prepare and extremely versatile. Pour it over zucchini noodles or a plate of spinach. If you have room for some extra carbohydrates, try spooning it over spaghetti squash.

INGREDIENTS | SERVES 4

1 pound cooked medium shrimp
¾ cup butter
2 cloves garlic, minced
1 tablespoon lemon juice

Benefits of Shrimp

Shrimp is an unusually concentrated source of the carotenoid astaxanthin, which acts as an antioxidant and an anti-inflammatory agent. Shrimp is also an excellent source of the mineral selenium.

1. Remove tails from shrimp. Set shrimp aside.

2. Melt butter in a large skillet over medium heat. When butter is hot, add garlic and sauté until translucent, 3–4 minutes. Add lemon juice and shrimp and cook over medium heat until shrimp is hot, about 2 minutes.

Creamy Chicken Zoodles

This recipe calls for zucchini noodles or zoodles, which you can easily make with a vegetable spiralizer. You can find a spiralizer at most home stores. If you prefer, you can also make zucchini noodles by julienning the zucchini with a vegetable peeler.

INGREDIENTS | SERVES 4

2 large zucchini

3 tablespoons extra-virgin olive oil

1 pound boneless, skinless chicken breast, cut into cubes

½ teaspoon salt

½ teaspoon black pepper

8 ounces fresh spinach

½ cup cream cheese

2 tablespoons grated Parmesan cheese

2 tablespoons feta cheese crumbles

1. Cut zucchini in long strips with a vegetable peeler or a spiralizer. Set zucchini aside on a paper towel and allow to sweat.

2. Heat olive oil in medium skillet over medium heat. Season chicken cubes with salt and pepper and add to hot pan. Cook chicken until no longer pink, about 10 minutes.

3. Remove chicken from pan with slotted spoon and set aside.

4. Add spinach to hot pan and sauté until wilted. Add cream cheese, Parmesan cheese, and feta cheese, and stir until melted. Add chicken back to pan and toss until coated. Remove from heat and pour over zucchini noodles.

"Spaghetti" and Spicy Meatballs

When you taste this recipe, you won't even miss regular pasta noodles. The zucchini has a mild flavor that serves as the perfect vehicle for the sauce and meatballs.

INGREDIENTS | SERVES 4

2 large zucchini
2 tablespoons extra-virgin olive oil
1 cup chopped white onion
2 cloves garlic, minced
1 large egg
¼ cup shredded pepper jack cheese
½ teaspoon salt
¼ teaspoon black pepper
⅛ teaspoon red pepper flakes
½ pound ground beef
½ pound ground pork
2 tablespoons butter
2 cups Marinara Sauce (see recipe in Chapter 9)

1. Preheat oven to 375°F.

2. Cut zucchini into long strips using a vegetable slicer or a spiralizer. Set aside onto a paper towel and allow to sweat.

3. Heat olive oil over medium-heat in a large skillet. Add onions and garlic and sauté until transparent, 3–4 minutes. Set aside and allow to cool.

4. Put egg, cheese, salt, black pepper, red pepper, beef, and pork in a large mixing bowl. Add onions and garlic and mix until evenly incorporated.

5. Shape meat mixture into 12 meatballs. Place meatballs on a baking sheet and bake for 20 minutes or until internal temperature reaches 165°F.

6. Put butter in a skillet and heat over medium heat. Add zucchini noodles and sauté, stirring frequently, until softened but still firm, about 5 minutes. Remove from heat.

7. Divide zucchini up into 4 servings. Top each serving with 3 meatballs and ½ cup marinara sauce.

Stuffed Pork Tenderloin

Pork is so versatile that you can use this recipe as a basic template and change the fillings to anything you want. Try ham instead of prosciutto or Gorgonzola cheese instead of feta.

INGREDIENTS | SERVES 4

1 pound pork tenderloin
4 slices prosciutto
4 slices cooked sugar-free bacon, chopped
½ teaspoon garlic powder
½ teaspoon ground sage
½ teaspoon black pepper
¼ teaspoon salt
½ teaspoon dry mustard
¼ cup cream cheese, softened
¼ cup feta cheese crumbles
1 cup frozen spinach, thawed
3 tablespoons extra-virgin olive oil

1. Preheat oven to 350°F.

2. Butterfly pork tenderloin and set aside.

3. Lay each slice of prosciutto down on the pork.

4. Put bacon, garlic powder, spices, cream cheese, feta cheese, and frozen spinach in a medium mixing bowl and beat until smooth.

5. Spread filling over prosciutto and roll tenderloin closed. Secure pork with a kitchen string.

6. Heat olive oil in a large pan over medium-high heat. Sear pork for 2 minutes on each side, then place in a baking dish.

7. Bake for 30 minutes or until inside is no longer pink and thermometer reads 160°F.

Zucchini Chicken Alfredo

This recipe calls for chicken, but the zucchini and Alfredo combination also goes well with shrimp.

INGREDIENTS | SERVES 4

2 large zucchini

½ teaspoon salt

½ teaspoon black pepper

¼ teaspoon paprika

¼ teaspoon garlic powder

1 pound boneless, skinless chicken thighs

2 tablespoons coconut oil

2 tablespoons butter

2 cups Alfredo Sauce (see recipe in Chapter 9)

Stocking Up on Chicken

Chicken thighs are regularly on sale because they are less popular than chicken breasts. Take advantage of these sales by buying several packages at a time and freezing them for later. You can even cook the chicken before freezing to save time when making recipes down the road.

1. Cut zucchini into long strips using vegetable peeler or spiralizer. Set aside on a paper towel and allow to sweat.

2. Sprinkle salt, black pepper, paprika, and garlic powder over chicken thighs. Heat coconut oil in a medium skillet over medium heat and place chicken in pan. Cook for 5 minutes, flip over, and then cook for another 5 minutes, or until no longer pink.

3. Remove chicken from heat with slotted spoon and chop into large pieces.

4. Add butter to hot pan. Once butter melts, add zucchini and sauté until softened but still firm, about 5 minutes. Add Alfredo sauce and chopped chicken to pan and toss until coated.

Pepperoni Meat-Za

Following a ketogenic diet doesn't mean that you have to give up pizza for good. Swap out the carbohydrate-filled crust for a crust made of meat and you're good to go.

INGREDIENTS | SERVES 4

1 pound ground beef

1 large egg

½ teaspoon garlic powder

½ teaspoon onion powder

½ teaspoon salt

½ teaspoon black pepper

1 teaspoon dried oregano

¼ cup grated Parmesan cheese

1½ cups Marinara Sauce (see recipe in Chapter 9)

1½ cups shredded mozzarella cheese

15 slices sugar-free pepperoni

1. Preheat oven to 400°F.

2. In a large mixing bowl, mix meat and egg together until combined. Add garlic powder, onion powder, salt, pepper, oregano, and Parmesan cheese and mix. Press meat mixture into a 9" pie plate, forming a pizza crust.

3. Bake for 20 minutes or until meat is no longer pink and thermometer reads 165°F. Remove from oven.

4. Spread marinara sauce evenly over cooked meat. Sprinkle mozzarella over sauce and top with pepperoni slices. Return to oven and bake until cheese is melted and bubbly, about 5 minutes.

Ground Pork Stir-Fry

You can change the flavor profile of this recipe by simply changing the spices you use. Use rosemary and thyme instead of garlic, onion, and sage.

INGREDIENTS | SERVES 4

2 tablespoons coconut oil

1 medium yellow onion

3 cloves garlic, minced

1 large zucchini

1 pound ground pork

1 (10-ounce) bag fresh spinach

1 cup chopped cooked broccoli

1 teaspoon ground sage

1 teaspoon granulated garlic

1 teaspoon granulated onion

1 teaspoon salt

1 teaspoon black pepper

½ teaspoon red pepper flakes (optional)

1 large avocado, diced

1. Heat coconut oil in a medium skillet over medium-high heat. Add onion and garlic and sauté until transparent, about 5 minutes.

2. Add zucchini and sauté until soft, another 3–4 minutes. Add ground pork and sauté until no longer pink. When meat is cooked, add spinach and sauté until wilted. Add broccoli, sage, granulated garlic, granulated onion, salt, black pepper, and red pepper flakes (if desired). Toss mixture until evenly covered with spices.

3. Remove from heat and divide into 4 bowls. Top each serving with ¼ avocado.

Take It Further

This recipe tastes even better when it sits overnight, as the flavors have more time to develop. Make it for dinner and heat it up in the morning—and put a fried egg on top to increase the fat and protein content.

Bacon-Wrapped Chicken

If you want really crispy bacon, you can partially cook the bacon before wrapping the chicken. This will help ensure that the bacon is thoroughly cooked by the time the chicken is.

INGREDIENTS | SERVES 4

1 pound (4 individual) boneless, skinless chicken breasts
1 cup cream cheese, softened
½ cup shredded pepper jack cheese
2 tablespoons dried chives
¼ teaspoon salt
¼ teaspoon black pepper
4 slices sugar-free bacon

1. Preheat oven to 400°F.

2. Cut a pocket into each chicken breast with a small paring knife. Set aside.

3. Put cream cheese, pepper jack cheese, chives, salt, and black pepper in a medium bowl and mix until combined.

4. Fill each chicken breast with ¼ of cream cheese mixture and wrap with 1 bacon strip. Secure with a toothpick.

5. Place chicken breasts in a baking pan and bake for 40 minutes or until a meat thermometer reads 165°F.

6. Turn oven to broil and broil on top rack until bacon is crispy, about 5 minutes.

Stuffed Green Peppers

You can swap the green peppers in this recipe for red peppers or yellow peppers if you prefer the taste, but keep in mind that this will change the carbohydrate count.

INGREDIENTS | SERVES 4

4 medium green bell peppers
1 tablespoon extra-virgin olive oil
½ cup chopped yellow onion
2 cloves garlic, minced
1 pound ground beef
4 slices cooked sugar-free bacon, diced
1 large tomato, diced
2 teaspoons Italian seasoning
¼ cup Marinara Sauce (see recipe in Chapter 9)
½ cup shredded mozzarella cheese
½ cup shredded Cheddar cheese

1. Preheat oven to 375°F.

2. Cut tops off of bell peppers and remove seeds. Set aside.

3. Heat olive oil in a large skillet over medium heat and sauté onion and garlic until transparent, about 5 minutes.

4. Add beef to skillet and cook until browned. Add bacon, tomato, and Italian seasoning and combine. Stir in marinara sauce.

5. Stuff each pepper with ¼ of meat mixture and stand peppers upright in a baking dish. Bake for 50 minutes or until meat reaches an internal temperature of 165°F.

6. Turn oven to broil and sprinkle cheese on top of meat mixture. Broil for 5 minutes or until cheese is melted and bubbly and peppers start to char. Remove from oven and serve hot.

Bunless Bacon Burgers

The combination of avocado and Homemade Mayonnaise in this recipe is so good you won't even miss the bun. For an even more decadent treat, add a fried egg on top.

INGREDIENTS | SERVES 4

1 pound 80/20 ground beef
⅓ cup heavy cream
⅛ teaspoon hot pepper sauce
1 clove garlic, minced
3 tablespoons chopped onion
¼ teaspoon black pepper
¼ teaspoon salt
4 slices American cheese
4 slices cooked sugar-free bacon
1 medium avocado, sliced
2 tablespoons Homemade Mayonnaise (see recipe in Chapter 9)

1. Turn oven on to broil.

2. Place beef in a large mixing bowl and add cream, hot sauce, garlic, onion, black pepper, and salt. Mix until combined.

3. Form into 4 patties and place on a broiling rack. Broil for 4 minutes on each side or until beef is no longer pink.

4. Top each burger with a slice of American cheese and leave under broiler for 1 more minute.

5. Remove from oven and top each burger with 1 slice bacon and ¼ sliced avocado. Drizzle ½ tablespoon mayonnaise onto each burger.

Shepherd's Pie

This recipe freezes very well, so save yourself some time by doubling the recipe and freezing half. You can use the frozen pie for dinner on a night that you don't feel like cooking.

INGREDIENTS | SERVES 6

2 tablespoons coconut oil

1 medium yellow onion, chopped

3 cloves garlic, minced

2 medium stalks celery, diced

1 medium zucchini, diced

1½ pounds ground lamb

1 teaspoon dried rosemary

1 teaspoon dried thyme

1 teaspoon black pepper

½ teaspoon salt

½ teaspoon garlic powder

4 cups cauliflower florets, boiled

¼ cup heavy cream

3 tablespoons butter

½ teaspoon garlic salt

¾ cup shredded Cheddar cheese

1. Preheat oven to 350°F.

2. Heat coconut oil in a large skillet over medium-high heat. When oil is hot, add onions and garlic and sauté until translucent, about 5 minutes. Add celery and zucchini and sauté until soft, another 5 minutes.

3. Add lamb, herbs, spices, and garlic powder and cook until no longer pink. Pour lamb mixture into a 9" × 13" baking dish.

4. Put boiled cauliflower, cream, butter, and garlic salt in a food processor and process until smooth. Pour cauliflower mixture on top of lamb. Top with cheese.

5. Bake until cheese is melted and pie is bubbly, about 25 minutes. Allow to cool for 10 minutes before serving.

Some Shepherd's Pie History

Shepherd's pie, which is also called cottage pie, was first developed in an attempt to use up leftover meat. Traditional shepherd's pie uses lamb. When beef is used instead of lamb, the same meal is called cottage pie.

CHAPTER 9

Soups, Dressings, and Sauces

Bacon Cheddar Soup

If you don't have an immersion blender, you can pour the soup into the pitcher of a regular blender instead. Just make sure that it's not too hot, or you may have an explosive mess on your hands.

INGREDIENTS | SERVES 4

4 slices thick-cut sugar-free bacon

1 small onion, chopped

2 cloves garlic, minced

3 cups cauliflower florets

½ teaspoon dry mustard

½ teaspoon black pepper

3 cups sugar-free chicken broth

2 cups heavy cream

2 cups shredded Cheddar cheese

1 tablespoon grated Parmesan cheese

Homemade Chicken Broth

You can easily make your own chicken broth by covering about 3 pounds of chicken bones with water in a slow cooker and letting it simmer on low for at least 12 hours. Many commercial chicken broths contain unhealthy ingredients and preservatives, and while homemade chicken broth doesn't last as long, it's better for you.

1. Cook bacon over medium-high heat in a medium skillet until crisp, about 10 minutes. Remove bacon from pan, reserving bacon grease. Return pan to heat.

2. Place onions and garlic in bacon grease and sauté until translucent, 3–4 minutes. Chop cauliflower florets into small pieces and add to onions and garlic. Sauté until tender, 7–10 minutes. Add dry mustard and black pepper and stir.

3. Transfer onions, garlic, cauliflower, and bacon grease to a large stock pot. Add chicken broth and heavy cream.

4. Stir all ingredients together and bring to a boil over medium heat. Once mixture begins to boil, reduce heat to a simmer.

5. Insert an immersion blender into the soup and blend until creamy. Add Cheddar cheese and Parmesan cheese and stir until melted.

6. Dice bacon and stir into soup. Serve hot.

Chilled Spicy Avocado Soup

Make this a satisfying vegetarian recipe by using vegetable broth in place of the chicken broth.

INGREDIENTS | SERVES 6

2 tablespoons olive oil

2 cloves garlic, minced

1 small white onion, diced

½ jalapeño, minced

3 large avocados, chopped

3 cups sugar-free chicken broth

¾ teaspoon black pepper

¼ cup fresh lemon juice

2 cups full-fat coconut cream

1. Heat olive oil in a small skillet. When oil is hot, add garlic, onion, and jalapeño and sauté until softened, 3–4 minutes. Remove from heat and allow to cool.

2. sAdd chopped avocados to a blender with chicken broth, black pepper, lemon juice, coconut cream, and onion and garlic mixture. Blend until smooth.

3. Refrigerate until chilled, about 4 hours. Serve cool.

Creamy Broccoli Soup

The creamy nutty flavor of the coconut milk in this recipe complements the broccoli nicely, but if you don't like the coconut flavor, you can use heavy cream instead.

INGREDIENTS | SERVES 6

2 tablespoons butter

2 stalks celery, diced

1 medium onion, diced

6 cups broccoli florets

½ teaspoon salt

½ teaspoon black pepper

4 cups sugar-free chicken broth

2 cups full-fat canned coconut milk

1. Heat butter over medium-high heat in a large stockpot. Add celery and onion and sauté until translucent, 3–4 minutes.

2. Add broccoli florets, salt, pepper, and chicken broth and bring to a simmer. Allow to simmer until broccoli is fork tender, about 10 minutes.

3. Add coconut milk and blend with an immersion blender until soup is smooth and creamy. Serve hot.

Be Choosy with Dairy

Heavy cream, cheese, and butter are staples on a ketogenic diet, but some dairy products are filled with hormones. Choose grass-fed butter, raw cheese, and organic heavy cream whenever possible.

Pumpkin Cream Soup

Instead of using cinnamon, nutmeg, and ginger in this recipe, you can use just over a teaspoon of pumpkin pie spice.

INGREDIENTS | SERVES 6

2 tablespoons coconut oil

2 tablespoons butter

¼ cup diced onion

2 cloves garlic, minced

3 cups sugar-free chicken broth

1½ cups pumpkin purée

½ teaspoon ground cinnamon

½ teaspoon ground nutmeg

⅛ teaspoon ground ginger

¼ teaspoon salt

¼ teaspoon black pepper

3 cups full-fat canned coconut milk

1. Heat coconut oil and butter in a stockpot over medium high heat. When oil and butter are hot, add onions and garlic and sauté until translucent, 3–4 minutes.

2. Add chicken broth, pumpkin purée, cinnamon, nutmeg, ginger, salt, and pepper and stir until combined.

3. Submerge an immersion blender into soup and blend until smooth and creamy. Allow to simmer for 20 minutes.

4. Stir in coconut milk. Serve hot.

Chicken Soup

Instead of canned chicken, you can use the meat from a precooked rotisserie chicken or poach a couple of chicken breasts and then shred them.

INGREDIENTS | SERVES 6

2 tablespoons olive oil

3 cloves garlic, minced

1 medium onion, diced

2 stalks celery, diced

4 ounces cream cheese

¾ cup heavy cream

1 (28.5-ounce) can shredded chicken breast

6 cups sugar-free chicken broth

1 teaspoon dried oregano

2 teaspoons Italian seasoning

2 bay leaves

¼ cup fresh chopped parsley

1. Heat olive oil in a large stockpot over medium-high heat. When oil is hot, add garlic and onions and sauté until translucent, 3–4 minutes. Add celery and sauté until soft, about 4 minutes.

2. Add cream cheese and heavy cream to pan and stir until cream cheese is melted.

3. Add remaining ingredients and bring to a boil. Once the soup starts boiling, reduce heat and allow to simmer for 25 minutes. Serve hot.

Marinara Sauce

Because this recipe freezes well, you can save yourself some time down the road by making a double batch and freezing what you don't use for later.

INGREDIENTS | MAKES 8 CUPS
(SERVES 16)

2 tablespoons butter

1 small yellow onion, minced

4 cloves garlic, minced

2 (28-ounce) cans crushed tomatoes

1 (14-ounce) can sugar-free tomato sauce

¼ cup extra-virgin olive oil

¼ cup red wine vinegar

2 tablespoons Italian seasoning

¼ cup chopped fresh parsley

¾ teaspoon salt

½ teaspoon black pepper

1. Heat butter in a large stockpot over medium-high heat. Add onions and garlic and sauté until browned, about 5 minutes.

2. Add crushed tomatoes, tomato sauce, olive oil, red wine vinegar, and seasonings. Stir and bring to a simmer.

3. Simmer for 45 minutes, stirring occasionally.

4. Serve immediately or store in the refrigerator in airtight container.

Let It Sit for a Bit

Tomato-based meals tend to develop better flavors after they sit for a day or two. For maximum flavor, make this sauce a couple of days before you need to use it and store it in the refrigerator.

Homemade Mayonnaise

You can use olive oil in this recipe in place of avocado oil. If you prefer a milder taste, opt for extra-light olive oil. If you like mayonnaise with a strong olive oil flavor, go for extra-virgin.

INGREDIENTS | MAKES 1¼ CUP (SERVES 10)

1 large egg, room temperature
Juice from ½ lemon, room temperature
½ teaspoon dry mustard
½ teaspoon salt
¼ teaspoon black pepper
1 cup avocado oil

Creating an Emulsion

Mayonnaise is made by creating an emulsion, or a mixture of oil and water (from the eggs). As you know, oil and water do not mix easily, so it's important to let the eggs and lemon juice reach room temperature before preparing this recipe. If you don't, the emulsion may fail and you'll be left with a runny mess.

1. Combine egg and lemon juice in a narrow container and let sit for 30 minutes.

2. Add dry mustard, salt, pepper, and avocado oil. Insert an immersion blender into mixture until it hits the bottom of the container.

3. Turn the blender on and blend for 30 seconds. As the mixture starts to emulsify, pull the blender out of the mixture slightly to mix in the oil on the top.

4. Transfer to a tightly sealed container and store in the refrigerator.

Garlic Aioli

This recipe calls for raw garlic, but if you prefer, you can sauté the garlic in a skillet with a small amount of olive oil before mixing.

INGREDIENTS | MAKES 1 CUP (SERVES 8)

1 cup Homemade Mayonnaise (see recipe in this chapter)

4 cloves garlic, minced

3 tablespoons olive oil

2 tablespoons fresh lemon juice

½ teaspoon salt

¼ teaspoon black pepper

1. Mix all ingredients together in a small bowl until smooth.

2. Cover and refrigerate before serving.

Hollandaise Sauce

If you prefer not to use the microwave, you can heat up the butter in a saucepan over low heat and then add it to the blender.

INGREDIENTS | MAKES 1 CUP (SERVES 4)

8 large egg yolks

¼ teaspoon salt

2 tablespoons fresh lemon juice

1 cup unsalted butter

Reduce Waste

Instead of throwing out the egg whites that you don't use in this recipe, scramble them up with some whole eggs and use them in a quiche or make the Bacon-Wrapped Egg Cups found in Chapter 6.

1. Put egg yolks, salt, and lemon juice in a blender and blend until smooth. Put butter in a microwave-safe dish and microwave until melted and hot, about 45–60 seconds.

2. With egg yolk mixture in blender, turn blender on low speed and slowly pour in the butter. The sauce will thicken.

Alfredo Sauce

You can replace the heavy cream in this recipe with 1 cup full-fat canned coconut milk, or use half heavy cream and half coconut milk.

INGREDIENTS | MAKES 1½ CUPS (SERVES 5)

½ cup butter

1 cup heavy cream

3 tablespoons grated Asiago cheese

3 tablespoons grated Parmesan cheese

½ teaspoon granulated garlic

¼ teaspoon ground nutmeg

¼ teaspoon salt

¼ teaspoon black pepper

1. Melt butter in a medium saucepan over medium heat. Add heavy cream and whisk for 2 minutes. Add Asiago cheese and Parmesan cheese and whisk until melted. Continue to cook for about 5 minutes, allowing mixture to simmer.

2. Stir in garlic, nutmeg, salt, and pepper. Remove from heat and serve immediately.

Avocado Basil Cream Sauce

Make this recipe only when you plan to use it right away. If you let it sit, the avocado tends to separate from the milk and cream.

INGREDIENTS | MAKES 1½ CUPS (12 SERVINGS)

1 large avocado
½ cup full-fat canned coconut milk
½ cup heavy cream
1½ tablespoons lemon juice
¼ cup chopped fresh basil
½ teaspoon salt
¼ teaspoon black pepper

Put all ingredients in a food processor or blender and process until smooth.

A Note on Herbs

You can substitute dried herbs for their fresh counterparts, but keep in mind that dried herbs are more concentrated so they have a stronger flavor. If you choose to use dried herbs instead of fresh, use only ⅓ of the fresh amount. For example, if the recipe calls for 3 tablespoons of fresh herbs, use only 1 tablespoon of dried herbs.

Blue Cheese Dressing

The dressing will thicken as it cools. You can thin it out by adding a little more white wine vinegar when you take it out of the fridge.

**INGREDIENTS | MAKES 1½ CUPS
(12 SERVINGS)**

⅓ cup Homemade Mayonnaise (see recipe in this chapter)

⅓ cup sour cream

⅓ cup heavy cream

1 tablespoon white wine vinegar

⅛ teaspoon garlic powder

¼ teaspoon salt

¼ teaspoon black pepper

⅓ cup blue cheese crumbles

Put mayonnaise, sour cream, heavy cream, and white wine vinegar in a small bowl and whisk until smooth. Stir in garlic powder, salt, and pepper. Fold in blue cheese crumbles. Refrigerate for at least 30 minutes before serving.

Ranch Dressing

You can easily add this dressing to salads, deli roll-ups, and chicken dishes for a quick boost in fat content.

INGREDIENTS | MAKES 1½ CUPS (12 SERVINGS)

1 cup Homemade Mayonnaise (see recipe in this chapter)

½ cup sour cream

½ teaspoon white vinegar

¼ cup chopped fresh parsley

2 tablespoons chopped fresh dill

½ teaspoon dried chives

¼ teaspoon garlic powder

¼ teaspoon onion powder

⅛ teaspoon salt

⅛ teaspoon black pepper

Put all ingredients in a mixing bowl and whisk until smooth. Cover and refrigerate for at least 30 minutes before serving.

Avocado Italian Dressing

You can make this more of a traditional Italian dressing by using light olive oil in place of avocado. Give it an Asian kick by using toasted sesame oil instead.

INGREDIENTS | MAKES 1½ CUPS
(SERVES 12)

1 cup avocado oil

¼ cup white wine vinegar

3 tablespoons water

1 teaspoon garlic salt

1 teaspoon onion powder

2 teaspoons dried oregano

½ teaspoon dried basil

1 teaspoon dried parsley

1 teaspoon salt

1 teaspoon black pepper

1. Whisk all ingredients together in a bowl until combined.

2. Serve immediately, or store at room temperature and shake or mix well before serving.

Storing It Safely

You can safely store this dressing at room temperature for several weeks. Put it in a sealable, leakproof container so that you can shake it vigorously to recombine ingredients before each use.

CHAPTER 10

Salads

BLT Salad

The combination of flavors in this bacon, lettuce, and tomato salad is so delicious that you won't even miss the bread.

INGREDIENTS | SERVES 4

1 pound sugar-free bacon

2 large tomatoes, diced

1 head romaine lettuce

2 large avocados, diced

½ cup Homemade Mayonnaise (see recipe in Chapter 9)

1 tablespoon white vinegar

Let it Sit

You can eat this salad as soon as it's chilled, or you can let it sit for a few hours or overnight to let the flavors develop. If you choose to let it sit overnight, leave the lettuce out and add it when you're ready to eat so that it stays crunchy.

1. Cook bacon over medium-high heat in a large skillet until crisp, about 10 minutes. Remove from heat, allow to cool, and then roughly chop and put in a medium mixing bowl.

2. Roughly chop romaine lettuce. Add lettuce, tomatoes, and avocado to bacon and toss until combined.

3. In a separate bowl, combine mayonnaise and white vinegar. Pour mayonnaise mixture over bacon mixture and toss to coat. Refrigerate until chilled, about 30 minutes. Serve chilled.

Bacon Spinach Salad with Creamy Ranch Dressing

You can use any high-fat dressing on this bacon spinach salad, but the dill in the ranch adds a nice flavor profile. Kick the fat up a notch by adding some avocado to the ranch dressing and blending until smooth.

INGREDIENTS | SERVES 4

1 (10-ounce) bag baby spinach
4 large hard-boiled eggs, peeled
8 slices sugar-free bacon, cooked
1 cup blue cheese crumbles
½ cup Ranch Dressing (see recipe in Chapter 9)

1. Put baby spinach in a large mixing bowl.

2. Roughly chop hard-boiled eggs and bacon and toss with spinach. Add blue cheese crumbles.

3. Top with ranch dressing and toss salad together. Serve immediately.

Eggs to Go

Hard-boiled eggs are a staple on the ketogenic diet. Boil one to two dozen at a time and store them in your refrigerator so you can use them on all your salads. Because they are so portable, hard-boiled eggs also make a great ketogenic diet snack.

Cobb Salad

This cobb salad is loaded with flavor and healthy fats. Switch it up a little bit by using blue cheese crumbles instead of feta and swapping out the ranch dressing for some homemade blue cheese.

INGREDIENTS | SERVES 4

8 cups chopped romaine lettuce

16 cherry tomatoes

1 cup diced sugar-free ham

4 large hard-boiled eggs, sliced

2 large avocados, diced

1 cup feta cheese crumbles

4 slices cooked sugar-free bacon, crumbled

½ cup Ranch Dressing (see recipe in Chapter 9)

1. Chop romaine lettuce and put in a large bowl. Cut cherry tomatoes in half lengthwise and put on top of lettuce. Add ham, eggs, avocados, feta cheese, and crumbled bacon. Toss to distribute.

2. Top with ranch dressing and toss until coated. Serve immediately.

Monkey Salad

Traditional monkey salad uses sliced bananas as a base, and that's where the "monkey" name comes from. Because bananas are high in carbohydrates, this version leaves them out, but the flavor is so good you won't miss them.

INGREDIENTS | SERVES 4

2 tablespoons butter

½ cup unsweetened coconut flakes

½ cup raw, unsalted cashews

½ cup raw, unsalted almonds

¼ cup 90% dark chocolate shavings

Sweet Treat

Monkey salad is the perfect sweet and satisfying treat. It's loaded with healthy fats that help keep you full between meals, and it's so easy to take on the go.

1. Melt butter in a medium skillet over medium heat. Add coconut flakes and sauté until lightly browned, 3–4 minutes.

2. Add cashews and almonds and sauté for 2 minutes. Remove from heat and sprinkle with dark chocolate shavings. Serve immediately.

Taco Salad

Being on a ketogenic diet doesn't mean you have to skip taco night. Ditch the shells for this salad and get the same delicious taco flavor without a great blood sugar spike.

INGREDIENTS | SERVES 4

2 tablespoons butter

1 pound ground beef

1 medium yellow onion, diced

1 (1-ounce) package sugar-free taco seasoning

1 head romaine lettuce, chopped

1 cup diced tomatoes

1½ cups shredded Cheddar cheese

½ cup Ranch Dressing (see recipe in Chapter 9)

½ cup salsa

½ cup sour cream

½ cup sliced black olives

1. Heat butter in a large skillet over medium-high heat. Add beef and onions and cook together until beef is no longer pink. Add taco seasoning to mixture and stir until evenly combined. Remove from heat and allow to cool.

2. Put chopped lettuce in a large mixing bowl. Add tomatoes, Cheddar cheese, beef mixture, and ranch dressing and toss until combined.

3. Divide up into 4 bowls and top each bowl with ⅛ cup of salsa, ⅛ cup of sour cream, and ⅛ cup of sliced olives.

Make Your Own Spice

Instead of using a prepared taco seasoning mix, which often contains sugar, artificial ingredients, and preservatives, make your own. Simply combine about 1 tablespoon of chili powder with about 1 teaspoon of cumin and about ¼ teaspoon of onion powder, garlic powder, oregano, salt, and pepper. You can adjust these proportions to your taste or add some red pepper flakes for a little kick.

Salmon and Avocado Salad

Instead of serving this as a salad, you can also spread the cream cheese mixture on each piece of smoked salmon and roll it up.

INGREDIENTS | SERVES 2

¼ cup cream cheese, softened
2 tablespoons extra-virgin olive oil
⅛ teaspoon salt
2 teaspoons lemon juice
8 ounces smoked salmon
2 large avocados, cubed

1. Put cream cheese, olive oil, salt, and lemon juice in a food processor or blender and process until smooth.

2. In a medium bowl, add smoked salmon to avocado and toss in cream cheese dressing. Refrigerate until chilled, 30 minutes to an hour. Serve chilled.

Spinach and Prosciutto Salad

The unsalted cashews in this recipe help satisfy that craving for something crunchy when you're eating a salad. As a bonus, they taste great with avocado.

INGREDIENTS | SERVES 4

8 cups baby spinach

12 ounces prosciutto

2 large avocados, diced

½ cup diced red onion

½ cup chopped raw, unsalted cashews

½ cup Avocado Italian Dressing (see recipe in Chapter 9)

1. Put spinach in a large mixing bowl. Dice prosciutto and put on top of spinach. Put diced avocado, red onion, and chopped cashews on top of spinach.

2. Add dressing to salad and toss to coat. Serve immediately.

Be Choosy with Nuts

When buying nuts, opt for raw, unsalted varieties rather than roasted, salted, or sugared versions. Raw nuts generally contain no added ingredients, while roasted, flavored nuts can contain unhealthy oils and sugar.

Gorgonzola Steak Salad

The combination of Gorgonzola crumbles and blue cheese dressing makes this salad taste like a decadent treat.

INGREDIENTS | SERVES 4

3 tablespoons olive oil

1 pound sirloin steak

1 teaspoon salt

1 teaspoon black pepper

8 cups mixed greens

4 large hard-boiled eggs, chopped

1 cup crumbled Gorgonzola cheese

½ cup Blue Cheese Dressing (see recipe in Chapter 9)

1. Heat olive oil in a large skillet over medium-high heat. While oil is heating, rub steak with salt and pepper. Place steak in hot skillet and cook until desired doneness, about 4 minutes on each side for medium-rare, 7 minutes on each side for medium, and 9 minutes on each side for well-done. Set aside and let rest for 10 minutes.

2. Put mixed greens in a large mixing bowl and top with hard-boiled eggs and crumbled Gorgonzola cheese.

3. Slice steak into thin strips and put on top of greens. Add dressing and toss until coated. Serve immediately.

Cheeseburger Salad

When you eat this salad, you get all the flavors of a cheeseburger without the insulin- and glucose-spiking bun.

INGREDIENTS | SERVES 4

1 pound ground beef

½ teaspoon salt

¼ teaspoon black pepper

⅓ cup sugar-free ketchup

1 tablespoon yellow mustard

1 teaspoon spicy brown mustard

1 head romaine lettuce

1 medium red onion, chopped

2 medium tomatoes, diced

4 dill pickle spears, cubed

1 cup shredded Cheddar cheese

½ cup Homemade Mayonnaise (see recipe in Chapter 9)

1 tablespoon white or apple cider vinegar

1. Brown ground beef in medium skillet over medium heat. Once beef is browned, add salt, pepper, ketchup, yellow mustard, and spicy mustard. Stir until combined. Remove from heat and set aside.

2. Chop romaine lettuce and put into a large mixing bowl. Top with onions, tomatoes, pickles, shredded cheese, and beef.

3. In a separate bowl, combine mayonnaise with vinegar and stir until smooth. Drizzle over salad and toss to coat. Serve immediately.

Spinach and Tuna Salad

You can swap out the tuna for chicken in this spinach and tuna salad or add hard-boiled eggs for some variations in taste. Make it spicy by adding a pinch of cayenne pepper.

INGREDIENTS | SERVES 2

2 (5-ounce) cans tuna

2 stalks celery, diced

¼ cup Homemade Mayonnaise (see recipe in Chapter 9)

4 cups spinach

4 slices sugar-free bacon, crumbled

1 large avocado, diced

2 tablespoons extra-virgin olive oil

Freshly ground black pepper

Mercury Concerns

If you're concerned about the mercury in tuna, keep in mind that adults can safely eat 18–24 ounces of tuna per month without a significant amount of mercury getting into their systems. If you'd like, swap out the tuna for canned salmon. Canned salmon is higher in omega-3 fatty acids and contains no mercury.

1. Combine tuna, celery, and mayonnaise in a small bowl and mix until combined.

2. In a large bowl, mix spinach, bacon crumbles, and avocado. Top with tuna mixture, drizzle with olive oil, and add freshly ground black pepper (if desired). Serve immediately.

Avocado Egg Salad

Instead of mashing the avocado into the salad along with the mayonnaise, you can cut it up it big chunks and toss it to cover with mayonnaise.

INGREDIENTS | SERVES 4

6 large hard-boiled eggs

¼ cup Homemade Mayonnaise (see recipe in Chapter 9)

½ avocado, chopped

½ teaspoon salt

¼ teaspoon black pepper

⅛ teaspoon crushed red pepper (optional)

1. Peel eggs and put into a medium mixing bowl. Mash eggs with a fork.

2. Add mayonnaise and avocado and continue to mash with a fork until combined. Stir in salt, black pepper, and red pepper, if desired.

Spinach, Feta, and Apple Salad

Granny Smith apples tend to be lower in sugar than sweeter varieties such as Pink Lady or Red Delicious. If you have some carbohydrates to spare and want a bit of a sweeter taste, swap the Granny Smith apple for another apple of your choice.

INGREDIENTS | SERVES 2

4 cups baby spinach

8 ounces cooked chicken, cubed

½ cup chopped red onion

½ cup crumbled feta cheese

½ small Granny Smith apple, diced

½ cup toasted pine nuts

¼ cup Ranch Dressing (see recipe in Chapter 9)

Combine all ingredients in a bowl and toss to coat. Serve immediately.

An Apple a Day

Apples are rich in quercetin and other flavonoids that slow digestion and help prevent a rapid spike in blood sugar levels. One cup of chopped apples contains 17 grams of carbohydrates, 13 of which come from natural sugars.

Chef Salad

Meat and cheese are the basis of a chef salad. Although this recipe calls for ham and turkey and Swiss and Cheddar, you can use any combination you'd like. Try adding roast beef and some pepper jack for a little kick.

INGREDIENTS | SERVES 4

8 cups chopped romaine lettuce

1 cup diced sugar-free ham

1 cup diced turkey

1 cup cubed Swiss cheese

1 cup cubed Cheddar cheese

4 large hard-boiled eggs, sliced

½ cup crumbled sugar-free bacon

½ cup Ranch or Blue Cheese Dressing (see recipes in Chapter 9)

Combine all ingredients in a large bowl and toss to combine. Serve immediately.

Kale and Salmon Salad

Baby kale is not as tough as regular kale, and it has a milder taste, too. If you're not a big kale lover, try baby kale before knocking it completely.

INGREDIENTS | SERVES 2

6 tablespoons olive oil, divided

2 cloves garlic, minced

8 ounces salmon fillet

½ teaspoon salt

¼ teaspoon black pepper

1 tablespoon lemon juice

4 cups chopped baby kale

1 large avocado, diced

2 tablespoons pine nuts

2 tablespoons apple cider vinegar

1. Heat 2 tablespoons olive oil in a large skillet over medium heat. Add garlic and sauté for 3 minutes.

2. Sprinkle salt and pepper over salmon and add to hot pan. Cook for 4 minutes on each side or until fish flakes easily with a fork. Drizzle lemon juice on top. Remove from heat.

3. Divide kale between two plates and top each plate with ½ avocado, 1 tablespoon pine nuts, and 4 ounces salmon.

4. In a separate bowl, combine remaining 4 tablespoons olive oil and apple cider vinegar. Pour half of mixture over each plate.

Bacon and Broccoli Salad

The longer this recipe sits, the better it gets, so make it the day before you plan to eat it for maximum flavor.

INGREDIENTS | SERVES 4

6 cups broccoli florets

8 slices cooked sugar-free bacon, crumbled

8 ounces sharp Cheddar, cubed

1 large avocado, diced

1 cup Homemade Mayonnaise (see recipe in Chapter 9)

2 tablespoons white vinegar

¼ teaspoon salt

¼ teaspoon black pepper

1. Combine raw broccoli, bacon, Cheddar cheese, and avocado in a large bowl.

2. In a separate bowl, combine mayonnaise, vinegar, salt, and pepper and stir until combined. Pour dressing over broccoli mixture and toss to coat. Refrigerate until chilled, about 30 minutes. Serve chilled.

Go Raw

Broccoli contains a high amount of sulforaphane, a compound that helps stimulate detoxification and may help reduce the risk for certain types of cancers. According to a report in the *Journal of Agricultural and Food Chemistry*, raw broccoli provides more sulforaphane than cooked broccoli, because the cooking process binds the compounds, making it less accessible.

CHAPTER 11

Side Dishes

Mashed Cauliflower

You can add more butter or cheese to this recipe if you need to increase the fat content so you can hit your fat goals for the day.

INGREDIENTS | SERVES 6

1 large head cauliflower
1 cup full-fat canned coconut milk
½ cup cream cheese, softened
¼ cup butter
½ teaspoon garlic salt
½ teaspoon salt
½ teaspoon black pepper

Smooth Operator

Using a food processor will make this mashed cauliflower perfectly smooth and creamy. If you prefer a chunkier version, use a handheld mixer instead and stop beating when the cauliflower has reached its desired consistency.

1. Break cauliflower into florets and steam in a double boiler until fork tender, about 8 minutes.

2. Remove from heat and transfer to a food processor. Add remaining ingredients and process until smooth.

Bacon-Wrapped Asparagus

Don't let the simplicity of this recipe fool you. These bacon-wrapped asparagus stalks are always a crowd pleaser.

INGREDIENTS | SERVES 4

12 asparagus spears, ends trimmed
6 slices sugar-free bacon

Help Insulin with Asparagus

Asparagus is loaded with chromium, a trace mineral that enhances the activity of insulin, helping the hormone deliver glucose more efficiently from the bloodstream into your cells.

1. Cut each strip of bacon in half lengthwise.

2. Wrap a piece of bacon around each asparagus spear and secure in place with a toothpick.

3. Grill over medium heat for 10 minutes, or until bacon is crisp, turning each spear over halfway through cooking time.

Creamed Brussels Sprouts

For a cheesier, gooier side dish, add ½ cup of shredded Cheddar cheese to these Brussels sprouts before you sprinkle on the pork rinds.

INGREDIENTS | SERVES 4

5 tablespoons butter, divided
2 cloves garlic, minced
2 cups sliced Brussels sprouts
¾ cup heavy cream
2 tablespoons grated Parmesan cheese
¼ teaspoon salt
¼ teaspoon black pepper
½ cup crushed pork rinds

1. Preheat oven to 350°F.

2. Heat 2 tablespoons butter in a medium skillet over medium-high heat. Add garlic and sauté for 3 minutes. Add Brussels sprouts and continue to sauté until Brussels sprouts are fork tender, about 5 minutes.

3. Transfer Brussels sprouts, garlic, and melted butter to a 9" × 9" baking dish. Add cream, Parmesan cheese, salt, and pepper. Sprinkle pork rinds evenly over the top of Brussels sprouts and top with remaining butter.

4. Cover and bake for 30 minutes. Serve hot.

Turnip Fries

Turnips are often overlooked at the supermarket, but they make a great alternative to carbohydrate-loaded potatoes when making fries.

INGREDIENTS | SERVES 2

2 large turnips, peeled and cut into 2" sticks

2 tablespoons olive oil

4 tablespoons grated Parmesan cheese

¼ teaspoon salt

¼ teaspoon black pepper

¼ teaspoon chili powder (optional)

1. Preheat oven to 425°F.

2. Place turnip sticks on foil-lined baking pan. Sprinkle olive oil, Parmesan cheese, salt, pepper, and chili powder (if desired) over turnips and toss to coat.

3. Spread out in a single layer. Bake in the oven for 15 minutes, flip fries over, and then bake for another 15 minutes. Serve warm.

Detox with Turnips

Pliny the Elder, a Roman philosopher, considered turnips to be one of the most important foods of his time. Turnips are cruciferous vegetables that are high in antioxidants and contain plant compounds called glucosinolates that help the liver process toxins.

Fried Cauliflower "Rice"

When shredding the cauliflower, process it just enough to create rice-like pieces, but not so much that it begins to blend together. If you process it too long, it will turn into mashed cauliflower.

INGREDIENTS | SERVES 6

1 large head cauliflower (about 6 cups)
2 tablespoons butter
2 tablespoons sesame oil
4 cloves garlic, minced
2 green onions, chopped
2 tablespoons coconut aminos
½ teaspoon garlic salt
3 large eggs, beaten
1 large avocado, sliced

1. Break cauliflower into florets and put through a food processor using the grating attachment.

2. In a large wok or skillet, heat butter and sesame oil. Add minced garlic and sauté on medium for 3 minutes.

3. Add cauliflower and sauté for another 5 minutes, stirring frequently, until cauliflower is softened. Add green onions, coconut aminos, garlic salt, and eggs and toss until eggs are cooked.

4. Top with sliced avocado.

Skip the Soy

Coconut aminos sauce is a soy-free seasoning alternative made from the sap of coconut blossoms that you can use in place of soy sauce in any of your recipes. There is absolutely no coconut flavor—it tastes just like soy sauce, but unlike soy sauce, which is highly processed and most likely contains GMOs, coconut aminos is GMO-free and contains 17 amino acids, vitamins, and minerals.

Roasted Broccoli with Parmesan

If you like your broccoli slightly charred, broil it for a few minutes before you take it out of the oven.

INGREDIENTS | SERVES 6

1 large head broccoli
2 tablespoons olive oil
2 cloves garlic, minced
¼ teaspoon salt
¼ teaspoon black pepper
¼ cup grated Parmesan cheese

Pre-Digested Protein

Parmesan cheese is aged so long that the proteins in it start to break down before it even hits your digestive system. Much of the protein in Parmesan cheese has already been broken down into peptides and free amino acids before you eat it. This makes digestion easier on you.

1. Preheat oven to 425°F.

2. Cut broccoli into bite-sized pieces and put onto a foil-lined baking sheet.

3. Drizzle olive oil on top of broccoli, add garlic, salt, and pepper, and toss to coat.

4. Spread out in a single layer and bake for 20 minutes, or until broccoli is tender. Add Parmesan cheese and bake for 5 more minutes, or until cheese is melted.

Bacon-Fried Cabbage

Cabbage comes in several varieties including green, red, and napa. For this recipe, you can use any type of cabbage you want. Cabbage newbies may want to go for green cabbage, which is milder in flavor.

INGREDIENTS | SERVES 4

8 slices sugar-free bacon

4 cups chopped cabbage

¼ cup chopped yellow onion

1 teaspoon garlic powder

1 teaspoon black pepper

½ teaspoon salt

1. Fry bacon in large skillet over medium-high heat until crispy, about 10 minutes. Remove bacon from heat and set aside. Allow to cool, then roughly chop.

2. Add chopped cabbage and chopped onion to hot bacon fat and sauté until cabbage is tender, about 8 minutes. Add garlic powder, black pepper, salt, and chopped bacon to cabbage and toss to combine.

Avocado and Cilantro Salad

The cilantro in this recipe imparts a clean flavor that gives this dish a wonderful Mexican quality.

INGREDIENTS | SERVES 4

4 medium avocados, diced

½ cup chopped cilantro

2 tablespoons lemon juice

2 tablespoons avocado oil or extra-virgin olive oil

½ small white onion, sliced thinly

½ cup crumbled feta cheese

½ teaspoon salt

½ teaspoon black pepper

⅛ cup sliced pickled jalapeño peppers (optional)

Combine all ingredients in a bowl and toss to coat.

Get Clean with Cilantro

Cilantro is highly noted for its ability to act as a natural cleansing agent. The chemical compounds in cilantro bind to toxic metals such as mercury and help remove them from the body. Cilantro also acts as a strong antioxidant and may reduce the risk of heart disease.

Buttery Garlic Spinach

This recipe calls for frozen spinach, but you can use fresh spinach in its place if you prefer.
Just thoroughly clean and chop the leaves before starting the recipe.

INGREDIENTS | SERVES 4

3 tablespoons butter

2 cloves garlic, minced

1 (10-ounce) package frozen spinach, thawed

¼ teaspoon garlic salt

¼ teaspoon black pepper

Heat butter in a skillet over medium-high heat. Add garlic and sauté for 3 minutes. Add spinach and stir until wilted. Toss with garlic salt and black pepper.

Cole Slaw

You can add this cole slaw to any meal to quickly increase its fat content.
Cole slaw goes especially well with bunless burgers.

INGREDIENTS | SERVES 8

¾ cup Homemade Mayonnaise (see recipe in Chapter 9)

¼ cup sour cream

2 tablespoons white vinegar

1 teaspoon celery salt

¼ teaspoon black pepper

2 tablespoons granulated erythritol

1 large head green cabbage, shredded

2 tablespoons chopped yellow onion

1. Combine mayonnaise, sour cream, vinegar, celery salt, black pepper, and granulated erythritol in a large bowl and whisk until combined and the granulated erythritol is dissolved.

2. Add cabbage and onion to bowl and toss until coated.

3. Refrigerate for 30 minutes. Serve chilled.

Cheesy Broccoli

Instead of using only broccoli, you can make this dish with a combination of broccoli and cauliflower for some variety.

INGREDIENTS | SERVES 4

6 cups broccoli florets, fresh or frozen
2 tablespoons extra-virgin olive oil
½ teaspoon salt
¼ teaspoon black pepper
2 tablespoons butter
1 cup heavy cream
1 cup shredded Cheddar cheese
2 tablespoons grated Asiago cheese
¼ teaspoon dry mustard

1. Preheat oven to 400°F.

2. Put broccoli florets on a foil-lined baking sheet and toss with olive oil, salt, and pepper. Bake for 25 minutes or until broccoli is fork tender.

3. While broccoli is cooking, melt butter in a medium saucepan over medium heat. Add cream and bring to a simmer. Reduce heat to low, add Cheddar cheese and Asiago cheese, and whisk until melted. Stir in dry mustard.

4. Remove from heat and pour over broccoli.

Garlicky Green Beans

Save time by buying a bag of green beans that has already been washed, cleaned, and trimmed for you.

INGREDIENTS | SERVES 4

1 pound green beans, trimmed
¼ cup butter
2 cloves garlic, minced
⅓ cup toasted pine nuts
¼ teaspoon salt
¼ teaspoon black pepper

Allicin and Allium

Like shallots, garlic belongs to the genus *Allium*, which also includes onions and leeks. The major compound in garlic, which is called allicin, is responsible for its smell as well as its health benefits, which include boosting the immune system, reducing blood pressure, and reducing the risk of Alzheimer's disease and dementia.

1. Bring large pot of water to a boil. Add green beans and cook until fork tender, 4–5 minutes.

2. Heat butter in a large skillet over medium heat. Add garlic and pine nuts and sauté for 3 minutes or until pine nuts are lightly browned.

3. Transfer green beans to skillet, add salt and pepper, and toss until coated.

Cheesy Bacon Brussels Sprouts

Brussels sprouts may be one of the most hated vegetables in America, but when you try them sautéed in bacon fat, they'll jump to the top of your list of favorites.

INGREDIENTS | SERVES 4

6 slices sugar-free bacon

1 pound Brussels sprouts, trimmed and cut in half lengthwise

1½ cups shredded pepper jack cheese

Benefits of Brussels Sprouts

Serving for serving, Brussels sprouts contain significantly more vitamin C than an orange. They're also rich in vitamin A, beta-carotene, folic acid, iron, magnesium, selenium, and fiber. Chinese medicine practitioners often recommend Brussels sprouts to help with digestive troubles.

1. Cook bacon in a large skillet over medium-high heat until crispy, about 10 minutes.

2. Remove bacon from pan and set aside. Add Brussels sprouts to hot pan and sauté until fork tender, about 8 minutes.

3. Chop bacon into small pieces and add to Brussels sprouts. Sprinkle cheese on top and stir until melted. Serve hot.

Creamed Spinach

The combination of Parmesan and Asiago cheeses gives this dish a strong Italian flavor that's sure to please a crowd.

INGREDIENTS | SERVES 4

4 tablespoons butter

3 cloves garlic, minced

¼ cup minced shallots

1 (10-ounce) package frozen spinach, thawed

½ cup heavy cream

½ cup grated Parmesan cheese

¼ cup grated Asiago cheese

½ teaspoon salt

¼ teaspoon black pepper

1. Heat butter over medium-high heat and add garlic and shallots. Sauté for 3 minutes. Add thawed and drained spinach and stir in heavy cream.

2. Stir in Parmesan and Asiago cheeses and continue stirring until melted. Season with salt and pepper. Serve hot.

Sweet Shallots

Shallots belong to the genus *Allium*, the same family that claims onions and garlic. They resemble onions, but their flavor is richer, sweeter, and more potent, so you need less of them when cooking. If you want to substitute onion for shallots in this recipe, double the amount of onion you use.

Mexican Cauliflower "Rice"

The fire-roasted tomatoes give this dish a slightly spicy, smoky flavor, but if you can't find them, you can use regular diced tomatoes in their place.

INGREDIENTS | SERVES 4

6 cups cauliflower florets
3 tablespoons butter
½ (14.5-ounce) can fire-roasted diced tomatoes
¼ cup chopped cilantro
1 large avocado, chopped
½ cup sour cream

1. Shred cauliflower with a food processor using the grating attachment.

2. Heat butter in a large skillet over medium-high heat and add shredded cauliflower. Sauté until tender, about 7–8 minutes. Add diced tomatoes and cilantro and stir until combined.

3. Divide into 4 servings and top each serving with ¼ chopped avocado and 2 tablespoons sour cream.

CHAPTER 12

Vegetarian

Peanut Butter Pancakes

If you want to switch it up, swap out the peanut butter in this recipe for cashew butter, almond butter, or sunflower seed butter.

INGREDIENTS | SERVES 4 (2 PANCAKES EACH)

½ cup cream cheese, softened

4 large eggs

⅓ cup unsweetened peanut butter

½ teaspoon vanilla extract

¼ teaspoon ground cinnamon

1 tablespoon coconut oil

1. Beat cream cheese, eggs, and peanut butter together in a medium mixing bowl. Stir in vanilla and cinnamon until mixture is smooth.

2. Melt coconut oil in a large skillet and pour ⅛ of the peanut butter mixture into the hot pan. Cook for 3–4 minutes and then flip. Cook for another 2–3 minutes. Repeat until all batter is cooked.

Cinnamon Noatmeal

This noatmeal provides the comfort of a hot bowl of oatmeal without all the carbohydrates or sugars found in boxed varieties.

INGREDIENTS | SERVES 4

3½ cups full-fat canned coconut milk

¼ cup cream cheese

⅔ cup flaxseed meal

⅔ cup chia seeds

⅔ cup shredded unsweetened coconut flakes

2 teaspoons ground cinnamon

½ teaspoon ground nutmeg

½ teaspoon vanilla extract

5 tablespoons granulated erythritol

1. Put coconut milk and cream cheese in a large saucepan and heat over medium heat until cream cheese is melted and mixture starts to simmer.

2. Turn heat to medium-low and add flaxseed meal, chia seeds, and coconut to saucepan. Stir until ingredients are mixed together. Add cinnamon, nutmeg, vanilla extract, and erythritol.

3. Serve hot.

Coconut Yogurt

A lot of commercial yogurts are full of sugar and artificial ingredients that almost completely negate any health benefits you'd get from them. It's easy to make your own yogurt at home with only two ingredients.

INGREDIENTS | SERVES 4

2 cans (13.5-ounce each) full-fat coconut milk

2 probiotic capsules

Picking a Probiotic

There are so many probiotics available that it can be difficult to know which one to pick. Choose a probiotic that contains at least seven different strains of bacteria and at least 5 billion organisms per dose. Make sure to store the probiotic per the manufacturer's instructions, as exposure to high heat and too much light can kill the bacteria, rending the probiotic useless.

1. Pour coconut milk into a blender. Open probiotic capsules and dump contents into blender. Blend until smooth.

2. Pour mixture into 4 separate sealable oven-safe containers. Seal containers and place on a baking sheet.

3. Put baking sheet with containers in the oven and turn oven light on. Keep the oven door closed and leave containers in the oven for 24 hours.

4. Store in the refrigerator for up to 7 days.

Veggie Omelet

This combination of eggs and veggies is the perfect pair for a ketogenic dieter. It provides quality fat and a good source of protein, and is loaded with vitamins and minerals.

INGREDIENTS | SERVES 4

2 tablespoons coconut oil
¼ cup chopped white onion
1 small zucchini, diced
¼ cup diced green pepper
2 cups fresh spinach
6 large eggs
¼ cup coconut cream
¼ teaspoon salt
¼ teaspoon black pepper
½ cup shredded Cheddar cheese
1 large avocado, chopped

1. Put coconut oil in a large skillet and heat over medium heat. When skillet is hot, add onions, zucchini, and green pepper. Sauté until soft, about 5 minutes. Add spinach and sauté until wilted.

2. Whisk eggs, coconut cream, salt, and pepper together in a medium bowl. Pour egg mixture over sautéed veggies and cook for 2–3 minutes, or until eggs begin to set. Lift the edges of the eggs with a spatula and tilt the skillet so that uncooked egg moves to the side of the pan. Continue cooking for about 3 minutes or until egg is almost fully set.

3. Add shredded cheese to half of the egg and flip the other side over with a spatula.

4. Let the omelet cook for 2–3 more minutes or until cheese is melted. Remove from heat and top with chopped avocado.

Crustless Quiche

Quiches are a ketogenic diet staple. They're easy to prepare and they store well, so you can make them in bulk and have a piece for breakfast all week.

INGREDIENTS | SERVES 8

12 large eggs

1 cup heavy cream

2 tablespoons olive oil

⅓ cup mushrooms

1 cup fresh spinach

¼ cup chopped white onions

½ cup chopped broccoli

1 teaspoon black pepper

½ teaspoon salt

½ teaspoon garlic powder

2 cups shredded Cheddar cheese

2 cups shredded Colby jack cheese

Make It "Muffins"

If you want to make this quiche more travel-friendly, pour an equal amount of the egg mixture into each well of a regular-sized muffin tin. You'll end up with 12 individual servings that you can just grab and go.

1. Preheat oven to 350°F.

2. Whisk eggs and heavy cream together in a medium bowl and set aside.

3. Heat olive oil in a medium skillet over medium-high heat and add veggies. Sauté veggies until soft and spinach is wilted, 3–4 minutes.

4. Add veggies, black pepper, salt, and garlic powder to egg mixture and whisk together.

5. Butter the bottom of a 9" × 13" baking pan and sprinkle 2 cups of cheese along bottom of pan. Pour egg mixture over cheese and sprinkle remaining cheese on top.

6. Bake for 25 minutes or until egg is set.

Tomato Cream Soup

Finish this recipe off with a dollop of sour cream, which, in addition to giving each spoonful a nice creamy texture, also ups the fat content.

INGREDIENTS | SERVES 4

½ cup butter
1 medium yellow onion, diced
2 cloves garlic, minced
1 (28-ounce) can whole peeled tomatoes
3 cups vegetable broth
1 cup full-fat coconut milk
¼ cup chopped fresh basil
¼ cup chopped fresh parsley
½ teaspoon salt
¼ teaspoon black pepper

1. Heat butter in a medium stockpot over medium-high heat. Add onion and garlic and sauté until translucent, 3–4 minutes.

2. Add remaining ingredients and stir until combined.

3. Insert an immersion blender and blend all ingredients together until smooth.

4. Turn heat to high and bring to a boil. Once soup starts boiling, reduce heat and allow to simmer for 30 minutes. Serve hot.

Stuffed Portobello Mushrooms

You can easily change the flavor of this recipe by using blue cheese, Gorgonzola cheese, or goat cheese in place of feta.

INGREDIENTS | SERVES 4

8 large portobello mushrooms
1 cup crumbled feta cheese
2 cups chopped fresh spinach
¼ cup chopped fresh oregano
2 tablespoons extra-virgin olive oil

The Power of Portobello

Portobello mushrooms are low in carbohydrates and loaded with essential vitamins and minerals, such as thiamine, magnesium, vitamin B$_6$, and iron, making them the perfect vehicle for getting quality sources of fat and protein.

1. Preheat oven to 350°F.

2. Remove stems from mushrooms and chop stems into small pieces. Put chopped stems, feta, spinach, and oregano in a medium bowl and toss to combine.

3. Brush each mushroom inside and out with olive oil and then stuff with feta mixture. Put on a baking rack and bake for 20 minutes or until mushroom is soft and cheese is melted.

Chocolate Chia Pudding

Chia pudding is so simple and versatile, you can make it with just about any combination of ingredients. Try sunflower butter in place of coconut butter and ½ cup brewed coffee in place of ½ cup of the coconut cream.

INGREDIENTS | SERVES 2

1 cup full-fat coconut cream

3 tablespoons unsweetened cocoa powder

2 tablespoons granulated erythritol

¼ cup coconut butter

3 tablespoons chia seeds

Ch-ch-ch-chia

A single ounce of chia seeds contains 9 grams of fat (5 of which are omega-3s) and 4 grams of protein. There are 12 grams of carbohydrates in an ounce, but since 11 of them come from fiber, an ounce of chia seeds clocks in at only 1 net carb, making them a ketogenic diet superfood.

1. Put all ingredients except chia seeds in a blender and blend until smooth.

2. Transfer to a sealable container and add chia seeds. Shake to combine.

3. Refrigerate for 8 hours or until chia seeds have absorbed enough liquid to turn mixture into a pudding-like consistency. Serve chilled.

Avocado and Walnut Salad

You can whip up this salad in a flash. Add a few cheese crumbles for a higher fat content.

INGREDIENTS | SERVES 6

2 medium limes

6 large avocados, cubed

2 cups walnut pieces

1 cup cherry tomatoes, halved

½ cup sliced black olives

1 tablespoon extra-virgin olive oil

¼ teaspoon salt

¼ teaspoon black pepper

In a bowl, squeeze juice from limes over avocados. Add remaining ingredients and toss until combined.

Wonderful Walnuts

Walnuts are loaded with protein, fiber, and a specific omega-3 fatty acid called alpha-linolenic acid, or ALA. Just ¼ cup of walnuts provides all the ALA you need for an entire day.

Coffee Coconut Berry Smoothie

For a different flavor, use blueberries or blackberries (or a combination of all three) in place of the raspberries.

INGREDIENTS | SERVES 2

1 cup full-fat canned coconut milk

1 cup brewed coffee

2 tablespoons unsweetened cocoa powder

¼ cup frozen raspberries

1 tablespoon granulated erythritol

2 tablespoons sugar-free cashew butter

Put all ingredients in a blender and blend until smooth.

Creamy Spaghetti Squash

If you want to reduce the carbohydrate count of this dish, replace the spaghetti squash with lightly sautéed zucchini noodles.

INGREDIENTS | SERVES 6

1 small spaghetti squash

3 tablespoons olive oil, divided

½ teaspoon salt

¾ cup cream cheese

¼ cup sour cream

½ cup full-fat canned coconut milk

½ cup heavy cream

⅓ cup grated Parmesan cheese

2 tablespoons grated Asiago cheese

½ teaspoon onion powder

1 teaspoon dried chives

Keep an Eye On It

Be careful not to overcook spaghetti squash. When you do, the flesh turns mushy and loses its spaghetti-like quality. Cook just until fork tender.

1. Preheat oven to 400°F.

2. Carefully cut spaghetti squash in half lengthwise and scoop out the seeds. Brush 2 tablespoons of olive oil over flesh of spaghetti squash and sprinkle salt on top. Place on baking pan, cut side up, and bake for 45 minutes or until squash is fork tender.

3. Scrape squash out of shell with a fork and put in a medium bowl.

4. Add remaining tablespoon of olive oil to a medium saucepan and heat over medium heat. Add cream cheese to saucepan and stir until melted. Add sour cream, coconut milk, heavy cream, cheeses, and onion powder to saucepan, stirring frequently until sauce is bubbling. Remove from heat and pour over spaghetti squash. Toss to coat. Sprinkle chives on top.

Cauliflower Casserole

If you prefer a thicker casserole, you can replace half of the sour cream in this recipe with equal parts softened cream cheese.

INGREDIENTS | SERVES 4

6 cups cauliflower florets
¼ cup heavy cream
2 tablespoons butter
¼ teaspoon garlic powder
¼ teaspoon onion powder
⅛ teaspoon paprika
½ teaspoon salt
¼ teaspoon black pepper
1½ cups shredded Cheddar cheese, divided
½ cup fire-roasted diced tomatoes
½ cup sour cream
2 tablespoons diced fresh jalapeños
½ cup sliced black olives

1. Preheat oven to 350°F.

2. Bring a large pot of water to a boil and add cauliflower florets. Boil until fork tender, about 8 minutes. Drain and transfer cauliflower to a food processor or blender. Add heavy cream, butter, garlic powder, onion powder, paprika, salt, and pepper and process until smooth. Add ½ cup of cheese and stir until combined.

3. Pour cauliflower mixture into a 9" × 9" baking pan and spread out evenly. Spread diced tomatoes on top of cauliflower and sour cream on top of tomatoes. Sprinkle with remaining cheese, jalapeños, and olives.

4. Bake for 45 minutes or until cheese is melted and casserole is bubbling. Allow to cool before serving.

Zoodles with Avocado Pesto

Traditionally, pesto is made with pine nuts, but for a different flavor you can replace the pine nuts with raw, unsalted walnuts.

INGREDIENTS | SERVES 4

4 large zucchini
2 medium avocados, divided
2 cups chopped fresh basil
1 tablespoon lemon juice
2 cloves garlic
½ cup plus 2 tablespoons extra-virgin olive oil, divided
½ teaspoon salt
¼ teaspoon black pepper
½ cup grated Parmesan cheese
½ cup pine nuts
1 cup kalamata olives

Show Olives Some Love

The monounsaturated fats found in olive have been shown to encourage weight loss by breaking down the fats inside your fat cells and reducing insulin sensitivity. At only 1 gram of carbohydrates for 5 olives, they are a perfect ketogenic diet treat.

1. Cut zucchini into long strips using a vegetable peeler or a spiralizer. Set zucchini "noodles" aside on a paper towel and allow them to sweat.

2. Peel 1 avocado, remove the pit, and scoop out flesh. Add avocado to a blender, along with basil, lemon juice, garlic, ½ cup olive oil, salt, black pepper, and Parmesan cheese.

3. Heat 2 tablespoons olive oil in a large skillet over medium heat. Add zucchini noodles and sauté until softened, but still firm, about 4 minutes. Pour sauce into skillet, along with pine nuts and kalamata olives, and toss to coat zucchini.

4. Remove from heat. Slice remaining avocado and add to zucchini mixture. Toss to combine.

Baked Zucchini

This baked zucchini dish gives traditional lasagna a run for its money. Increase its nutritional content by adding some mushrooms and sautéed spinach.

INGREDIENTS | SERVES 4

2 tablespoons extra-virgin olive oil

½ cup chopped yellow onion

4 medium zucchini, julienned

1½ cups shredded mozzarella cheese, divided

½ cup full-fat ricotta cheese

2 tablespoons cream cheese, diced

1¼ cups Marinara Sauce (see recipe in Chapter 9)

2 cloves garlic, minced

¼ cup chopped fresh basil

¼ cup chopped fresh oregano

½ teaspoon salt

½ teaspoon black pepper

1. Preheat oven to 350°F.

2. Heat olive oil in a large skillet over medium heat and add onion. Sauté until translucent, about 3 minutes, then add zucchini. Sauté for another 4 minutes or until zucchini is softened, but still firm.

3. Add ½ cup mozzarella cheese, ricotta cheese, cream cheese, marinara, garlic, basil, oregano, salt, and pepper to the pan. Bring to a simmer and remove from heat once cream cheese is melted.

4. Transfer to an 8" × 8" baking dish. Top with remaining mozzarella and bake for 15 minutes or until cheese is melted and casserole is bubbling.

Ricotta-Stuffed Eggplant

The best eggplants are those that are firm and shiny without any broken skin. Smaller eggplants also tend to be less bitter than larger ones, so keep that in mind when choosing eggplants for this recipe.

INGREDIENTS | SERVES 4

2 small eggplants

¼ cup extra-virgin olive oil, divided

½ teaspoon salt

¼ teaspoon black pepper

2 cloves garlic, minced

2 tablespoons minced shallots

1 (8-ounce) container full-fat ricotta cheese

½ cup shredded mozzarella cheese

Male versus Female

Did you know that there are male and female eggplants? The male eggplants have fewer seeds than the female eggplants, so they tend to be less bitter. You can determine the sex of an eggplant by looking at the indentation on the bottom. If the indentation is shallow and round, it's a male; if the indentation is deep and more rectangular, it's a female.

1. Preheat oven to 350°F.

2. Cut eggplants in half and scoop out some of the insides to create a bowl. Brush bowls with 2 tablespoons of olive oil and sprinkle with salt and pepper. Dice insides and set aside.

3. Place eggplant halves on a baking sheet, cut side up, and bake for 20 minutes or until eggplant is soft.

4. While eggplant is baking, heat up remaining olive oil in a skillet over medium heat. Add chopped eggplant, garlic, and shallots to pan and sauté until soft, about 8 minutes. Remove from heat and allow to cool slightly.

5. Combine cooked eggplant, ricotta, and mozzarella cheese in a bowl. When eggplants are done cooking, fill them with cheese mixture, and return to the oven for 10 minutes or until cheese is melted and bubbly.

CHAPTER 13

Snacks

Deviled Eggs

Deviled eggs are a staple at any party, and they make the perfect ketogenic diet snack. Whip some up and store them in your refrigerator for when you need some fat and protein in a hurry.

INGREDIENTS | SERVES 6

6 large hard-boiled eggs

¼ cup Homemade Mayonnaise (see recipe in Chapter 9)

1 teaspoon white vinegar

1 teaspoon dry mustard

½ teaspoon salt

¼ teaspoon black pepper

⅛ teaspoon smoked paprika

1. Peel eggs and cut in half lengthwise. Scoop out egg yolks and put in a small mixing bowl.

2. Mash yolks with a fork, then add mayonnaise, vinegar, mustard, salt, and pepper. Continue to mash until combined.

3. Divide mixture into 12 equal portions and fill each egg white half. Sprinkle with paprika.

Pizza Bites

You won't even miss the crust when you try these pizza bites.
And the best part? They're ready to go in under 5 minutes.

INGREDIENTS | SERVES 6

24 slices sugar-free pepperoni

½ cup Marinara Sauce (see recipe in Chapter 9), divided

½ cup shredded mozzarella cheese

1. Turn on oven broiler.

2. Line a baking sheet with parchment paper and put pepperoni slices in a single layer on baking sheet.

3. Put 1 teaspoon of marinara sauce on each pepperoni slice and spread out with a spoon. Add 1 teaspoon of cheese on top of marinara.

4. Put baking sheet in the oven and broil for 3 minutes or until cheese is melted and slightly brown.

5. Remove from baking sheet and transfer to a paper towel–lined baking sheet to absorb excess grease.

Prosciutto Chips

These prosciutto chips are so simple and delicious, you'll wonder why you never thought of them before. All you need is some prosciutto and an oven.

INGREDIENTS | SERVES 4

12 ounces (12 slices) of prosciutto

A Little about Prosciutto

Prosciutto is made from the hind leg of a pig, or the ham. It is sliced thinly and rubbed with salt, which draws out the moisture to concentrate the flavor. This process, called curing, can take a few months to several years.

1. Preheat oven to 350°F.

2. Line a baking sheet with parchment paper and lay prosciutto slices out in a single layer. Bake for 12 minutes, or until prosciutto is crispy.

3. Let cool completely before eating.

Stuffed Olives

You can use any type of olive you want for this recipe, but green olives have a tangy flavor that complements the blue cheese wonderfully.

INGREDIENTS | SERVES 8

¼ cup blue cheese crumbles
¼ cup cream cheese, softened
24 large green olives

1. Beat blue cheese and cream cheese together in a small bowl until light and fluffy.

2. Fill each olive with 1 teaspoon filling. Serve at room temperature.

Bacon-Wrapped Chicken Bites

Serve these bacon-wrapped chicken bites with a side of Ranch Dressing (see recipe in Chapter 9) to increase both the flavor and the fat content.

INGREDIENTS | SERVES 6

12 ounces boneless, skinless chicken breast
½ teaspoon salt
½ teaspoon black pepper
5 slices sugar-free bacon

1. Preheat oven to 375°F.

2. Cut chicken into 1" cubes and toss with salt and pepper.

3. Cut each slice of bacon into 3 pieces and wrap each piece of chicken in a piece of bacon. Secure with a toothpick.

4. Put wrapped chicken on a broiler rack and bake for 30 minutes, turning over halfway through cooking. Turn oven to broil and broil for 3–4 minutes or until bacon is crispy.

Jalapeño Poppers

To double the yield of this recipe, cut the jalapeños in half and wrap each half in a half piece of bacon.

INGREDIENTS | SERVES 4

8 jalapeño peppers
½ cup cream cheese, softened
½ cup shredded pepper jack cheese
8 slices sugar-free bacon

Turn Up the Heat

The capsaicin in chili peppers is thermogenic, which means it generates heat by increasing the metabolism of adipose, or fat, tissue. Eating capsaicin-rich foods may help stimulate the body's ability to burn fat.

1. Preheat oven to 425°F.

2. Cut about ⅓ of each pepper off lengthwise to make a little pocket for filling. Scoop out seeds.

3. Mix cream cheese and pepper jack cheese together in a small bowl. Divide filling into 8 equal portions and stuff each pepper with cheese filling.

4. Wrap each pepper in bacon. Lay flat on a cookie sheet lined with aluminum foil and bake for 15–20 minutes, or until bacon is crispy.

Pumpkin Pie Coconut Crisps

The possibilities for this recipe are endless. You can experiment with any combination of spices you want. Make them sweet or savory or a combination of both.

INGREDIENTS | SERVES 4

2 tablespoons coconut oil
½ teaspoon vanilla extract
½ teaspoon pumpkin pie spice
1 tablespoon granulated erythritol
2 cups unsweetened coconut flakes
⅛ teaspoon salt

Cuckoo for Coconuts

Coconuts are rich in a specific type of fat called medium-chain triglycerides (MCTs). Instead of circulating through the blood like other fats, MCTs go straight to the liver where they're burned for energy. Because your body doesn't store MCTs, eating them can help boost weight loss.

1. Preheat oven to 350°F.

2. Put coconut oil in a microwave-safe bowl and microwave until melted, about 20 seconds. Add vanilla extract, pumpkin pie spice, and granulated erythritol to coconut oil and stir until combined.

3. Pour coconut oil mixture over coconut flakes and toss to coat. Spread out in a single layer on a cookie sheet and sprinkle with salt.

4. Bake for 5 minutes or until coconut is crispy.

Pepperoni Chips

Make sure to thoroughly blot away the excess grease in this recipe. If you don't you'll end up with soggy chips instead of crispy ones.

INGREDIENTS | SERVES 4

24 sugar-free pepperoni slices

1. Preheat oven to 425°F.

2. Line a baking sheet with parchment paper and lay out pepperoni slices in a single layer.

3. Bake for 10 minutes and then remove from oven and use a paper towel to blot away excess grease. Return to the oven for 5 minutes or until pepperoni is crispy.

Guacamole

Guacamole is a ketogenic diet staple. Eat it with some celery stalks, put it on top of your taco bowls, or spoon it right out of the bowl.

INGREDIENTS | SERVES 4

3 large avocados

Juice from 1 lime

2 large Roma tomatoes, diced

2 cloves garlic, minced

¼ cup chopped fresh cilantro

¼ cup chopped red onion

½ teaspoon salt

½ teaspoon black pepper

1 tablespoon diced jalapeño (optional)

1. Cut avocados in half lengthwise, remove the pit, and scoop them out of the skin and into a medium bowl. Add lime juice. Use a fork to mash avocado and lime together, leaving some chunks intact.

2. Add tomatoes, garlic, cilantro, onion, salt, pepper, and jalapeño (if desired). Mash with a fork until combined.

Amazing Avocado

About 77 percent of the calories in avocados come from fat, which makes it one of the fattiest foods in the world. Ounce for ounce avocados also contain more potassium than bananas, so they're especially beneficial during the initial stages of a ketogenic diet when you're losing water weight and electrolytes.

Parmesan Chips

You can make this recipe with any type—or combination of types—of cheeses you want. Try Cheddar, pepper jack, or a combination of Parmesan and Cheddar.

INGREDIENTS | SERVES 4 (MAKES 16 CHIPS)

½ cup grated Parmesan cheese
½ cup shredded Parmesan cheese

1. Preheat oven to 375°F.

2. Mix grated and shredded Parmesan cheese together. Drop by the tablespoon onto parchment paper–lined baking sheets.

3. Bake for 5 minutes or until cheese is crisp and slightly browned.

4. Remove from oven and allow to cool. Peel chips off parchment paper and serve.

Tuna Salad and Cucumber Bites

These bites are an easy snack that's good on the go.
Give yourself a little variety by using canned chicken or canned salmon in place of tuna.

INGREDIENTS | SERVES 4

1 medium cucumber

2 (5-ounce) cans of tuna

2 large hard-boiled eggs, peeled and chopped

½ cup Homemade Mayonnaise (see recipe in Chapter 9)

½ teaspoon salt

½ teaspoon black pepper

2 teaspoons goat cheese

Cool As a Cucumber

Cucumbers are 96 percent water, so they not only provide a good vehicle for getting in your protein and fat but also help keep you hydrated. The water in cucumber helps flush out toxins as well.

1. Wash and cut cucumber into rounds.

2. Drain tuna and put in a medium bowl with chopped eggs, mayonnaise, salt, and pepper. Mash with a fork until combined.

3. Spread an equal amount of goat cheese on each cucumber slice and top with tuna salad mixture.

Green Deviled Eggs

Adding avocado to traditional deviled eggs provides a healthy dose of monounsaturated fats and increases vitamin K, folate, vitamin C, and potassium content.

INGREDIENTS | SERVES 2

4 large hard-boiled eggs

1 large avocado, chopped

¼ cup Homemade Mayonnaise (see recipe in Chapter 9)

1 teaspoon lime juice

1 tablespoon feta cheese

2 teaspoons light olive oil

⅛ teaspoon salt

¼ teaspoon black pepper

1. Peel hard-boiled eggs and cut in half lengthwise. Scoop out yolks and place in a small bowl.

2. Put remaining ingredients in bowl with egg yolks and mash with a fork until combined.

3. Fill each egg white half with an equal amount of the yolk mixture. Sprinkle pepper on top.

Bacon-Wrapped Avocado Bites

The combination of bacon and avocado may not sound like a good combination, but don't knock it 'til you try it: the salty, crispy bacon and smooth, creamy avocado make the perfect pair.

INGREDIENTS | SERVES 4

2 large avocados
8 slices of sugar-free bacon
½ teaspoon garlic salt

Precook Your Bacon

If you cook avocado too long, the avocado can turn bitter. To avoid this, you can shorten the cooking time of this recipe by slightly precooking the bacon—enough that it's partially cooked but still bendable—and then wrapping it around the avocado and putting it in the oven.

1. Preheat oven to 425°F.

2. Cut each avocado into 8 equal-sized slices, making 16 slices total.

3. Cut each piece of bacon in half. Wrap each half slice of bacon around each piece of avocado.

4. Place avocado on parchment-lined cookie sheet and bake for 15 minutes. Turn oven to broil and continue to cook for another 2–3 minutes until bacon becomes crispy.

Pepperoni Cheese Bites

Enjoy this recipe cold or put each pepperoni bite in the oven just until the cheese melts for a warm, tasty treat.

INGREDIENTS | SERVES 2

4 sticks mozzarella string cheese
16 slices sugar-free pepperoni

1. Cut each string cheese into 4 equal pieces.

2. Wrap each piece in a slice of pepperoni and secure with a toothpick.

Chocolate Mousse

You'll love this mousse so much you won't even miss the real thing. The avocado adds healthy fats, but the taste is camouflaged by the cocoa powder.

INGREDIENTS | SERVES 4

½ cup cream cheese, softened

½ cup butter, softened

2 tablespoons granulated erythritol

½ large avocado

2 tablespoons unsweetened cocoa powder

⅔ cup heavy cream

1. Beat cream cheese, butter, and granulated erythritol together in a medium bowl until light and fluffy.

2. Add avocado and cocoa powder and beat until smooth. Stir in heavy cream.

3. Divide into 4 serving dishes and refrigerate until chilled, about 30 minutes. Serve cold.

Whip Up Some Cream

You can turn this from a snack into dessert by whipping up some coconut cream to put on top. Simply take the coconut cream from a can of coconut milk that's been refrigerated for 24 hours, add a couple of tablespoons of powdered erythritol and a teaspoon of vanilla extract, and beat for 2 to 4 minutes, or until cream is light and fluffy.

CHAPTER 14

Desserts

Pecan-Crusted Cheesecake

The pecan crust in this cheesecake is so good, you'll wonder why you ever made it with graham crackers.

INGREDIENTS | SERVES 12

1 cup pecans

½ cup butter

¾ cup almond meal

½ teaspoon ground cinnamon

1¼ cup erythritol powdered sweetener, divided

16 ounces cream cheese, room temperature

1 cup sour cream, room temperature

4 large eggs, room temperature

2 teaspoons vanilla extract

1 teaspoon lemon juice

½ teaspoon lemon zest

Powerful Pecans

Pecans are one of the most antioxidant-rich tree nuts. They also contain more than 19 vitamins and minerals, including vitamin A, folic acid, magnesium, potassium, and zinc.

1. Preheat oven to 375°F.

2. Place pecans in a food processor and pulse until pecans are crushed.

3. Melt butter in medium saucepan. Add crushed pecans, almond meal, cinnamon, and ¼ cup erythritol to melted butter. Stir until combined.

4. Allow mixture to cool slightly and pour into a 9" pie plate. Press mixture into pie plate so the bottom and sides are adequately covered.

5. Bake in oven until slightly browned, about 10 minutes.

6. Reduce oven temperature to 325°F.

7. Put cream cheese in a stand mixer and beat until fluffy, about 2 minutes.

8. Add sour cream to cream cheese and beat until incorporated.

9. Add eggs, vanilla, lemon juice, lemon zest, and remaining 1 cup erythritol and beat until smooth.

10. Pour cream cheese mixture on top of pecan crust.

11. Bake for 45 minutes. Cake should still jiggle when you remove it from the oven.

12. Allow to cool, then store in the refrigerator until ready to serve.

Chocolate Brownie Cheesecake

Throw a handful or two of nuts into this recipe to increase the unsaturated fat content and make this dessert even more nutritious.

INGREDIENTS | SERVES 12

4 ounces unsweetened chocolate
½ cup butter
4 large eggs, divided
2¼ cups granulated erythritol, divided
1 teaspoon vanilla extract
½ cup almond flour
½ teaspoon salt
16 ounces cream cheese
¼ cup sour cream
¼ cup full-fat canned coconut milk
½ teaspoon vanilla extract

1. Preheat oven to 325°F.

2. Melt chocolate and butter together in a medium saucepan over low heat.

3. In a large bowl, beat 2 eggs, 1½ cups granulated erythritol, and vanilla extract until combined. Add almond flour and salt. Beat until incorporated. Add chocolate and butter mixture and beat until smooth.

4. Pour brownie mixture into the bottom of a greased 9" springform pan.

5. Bake for 20 minutes, or until a knife inserted in the center of the brownies comes out clean.

6. Beat cream cheese in a stand mixer until fluffy, about 2 minutes.

7. Add sour cream and coconut milk and beat until incorporated. Beat in remaining 2 eggs, remaining ¾ cup granulated erythritol, and vanilla extract.

8. Pour cream cheese mixture over brownie mixture.

9. Reduce oven temperature to 300°F and bake for 45 minutes. Let cool and store in refrigerator until ready to serve.

Lemon Mug Cake with Lemon Icing

Don't skip the zest in this recipe! The small amount of lemon zest really enhances the lemony flavor.

INGREDIENTS | SERVES 2

¾ cup almond flour

3 tablespoons granulated erythritol

½ teaspoon baking powder

⅛ teaspoon salt

Juice and zest of 1 lemon

1 large egg

2 tablespoons butter, melted

2 tablespoons powdered erythritol

½ teaspoon water

½ teaspoon lemon juice

Zest Away

When zesting a lemon, remove only the yellow outer skin. The white part just under the yellow skin has a bitter taste that can be unpleasant. A special kitchen tool called a microplane is available to help make zesting easier.

1. In a medium bowl, mix almond flour, granulated erythritol, baking powder, and salt together. Add lemon juice, lemon zest, egg, and melted butter and whisk until combined.

2. In a small bowl, mix powdered erythritol, water, and lemon juice together.

3. Divide almond flour mixture evenly between 2 microwave-safe mugs.

4. Microwave for 90 seconds each.

5. Drizzle icing mixture on top of each mug cake. Serve warm.

Chocolate Mug Cake

This chocolate mug cake is a great way to have a chocolate treat without having to make an entire batch of brownies.

INGREDIENTS | SERVES 2

2 tablespoons butter, melted

3 tablespoons almond flour

1 tablespoon coconut flour

1 large egg

2 tablespoons granulated erythritol

¼ teaspoon vanilla extract

⅛ teaspoon salt

¾ teaspoon baking powder

1½ tablespoons unsweetened cocoa powder

1. Put all ingredients in a small bowl and whisk until smooth.

2. Split the batter evenly between two microwave-safe mugs.

3. Microwave each mug for 75 seconds or until batter has set.

Peanut Butter Cookies

Give these cookies a crunch by using crunchy peanut butter instead of creamy peanut butter or by adding a few handfuls of chopped peanuts.

INGREDIENTS | SERVES 18

1 cup sugar-free peanut butter
¼ cup butter, softened
1 cup granulated erythritol
1 large egg, lightly beaten
1 teaspoon vanilla extract
½ teaspoon baking soda
¼ teaspoon sea salt

1. Preheat oven to 350°F.

2. In a medium-sized bowl, beat together peanut butter and butter until combined and fluffy.

3. Add granulated erythritol, egg, and vanilla extract and mix until combined.

4. Stir in baking soda and salt.

5. Drop by tablespoonfuls onto an ungreased cookie sheet.

6. Bake for 10 minutes, or until lightly browned.

Chocolate Ice Cream

This recipe calls for the use of an ice-cream maker, but not having one isn't a deal-breaker. Instead of using an ice-cream maker, you can stir the mixture in the bowl every 30–45 minutes while it cools in the refrigerator.

INGREDIENTS | SERVES 4

1 large ripe avocado

1 cup full-fat canned coconut milk

1 cup heavy cream

1 teaspoon vanilla extract

1 cup unsweetened cocoa powder

1 cup granulated erythritol

Make It Your Own

This is a basic chocolate ice cream recipe that you can make your own by adding your own mix-ins. Try unsweetened coconut flakes, dark chocolate shavings, or chopped peanuts.

1. Cut avocado in half and scoop out contents into a medium bowl. Add coconut milk, heavy cream, and vanilla extract to the bowl. Beat mixture until smooth.

2. Add cocoa powder and granulated erythritol and beat until smooth.

3. Store in a metal bowl in the refrigerator for 6–12 hours, then put mixture into an ice-cream maker, following manufacturer's instructions for use.

4. Serve immediately or store in the freezer until ready to serve.

Snickerdoodle Cookies

Change the flavor of these cookies by rolling them in pumpkin pie spice instead of cinnamon before cooking.

INGREDIENTS | SERVES 12

1½ cups almond flour
¼ teaspoon baking soda
⅛ teaspoon salt
½ cup butter, softened
1 cup plus 2 tablespoons granulated erythritol, divided
1 large egg
1 teaspoon vanilla extract
1 teaspoon ground cinnamon

1. Preheat oven to 350°F.

2. Mix together almond flour, baking soda, and salt in a small mixing bowl.

3. In a separate bowl, beat butter and 1 cup granulated erythritol together until light and fluffy, about 2 minutes. Beat in egg and vanilla.

4. Stir in almond flour mixture.

5. In a separate bowl, mix remaining 2 tablespoons granulated erythritol with cinnamon.

6. Roll dough into 12 balls. Roll balls in cinnamon mixture and place on an ungreased baking sheet.

7. Press down on balls with the palm of your hand or the bottom of a glass to flatten them.

8. Bake for 8 minutes, or until slightly browned.

Chocolate Brownies

If you have some calories to spare, top these chocolate brownies with homemade chocolate ice cream and some whipped coconut cream for a decadent sundae.

INGREDIENTS | SERVES 12

1 cup almond flour
4 tablespoons unsweetened cocoa powder
½ teaspoon baking powder
¼ teaspoon salt
¾ cup granulated erythritol
½ cup butter, melted
3 large eggs
1 teaspoon vanilla extract

1. Preheat oven to 350°F.

2. Mix almond flour, cocoa powder, baking powder, and salt in a small bowl.

3. In a medium bowl, beat granulated erythritol and butter together. Beat in eggs, one at a time, and vanilla.

4. Stir dry ingredients into butter mixture.

5. Pour batter into a greased 8" × 8" baking pan. Bake for 30 minutes, or until a toothpick inserted in the center comes out clean.

Chocolate Fudge Sauce

This is the perfect chocolate fudge sauce to top off any of your desserts. You can even add it to some full-fat coconut milk and blend for a chocolate milk shake.

INGREDIENTS | SERVES 8

4 ounces cream cheese, softened

4 ounces unsweetened baking chocolate

⅓ cup powdered erythritol

¼ cup heavy cream

½ teaspoon vanilla extract

1. Melt cream cheese and baking chocolate in a double boiler over medium heat, stirring frequently until smooth.

2. Add erythritol and heavy cream and whisk until smooth.

3. Remove from heat and stir in vanilla extract.

4. Serve warm.

Pistachio Pudding

After you try this homemade pistachio pudding, you will never look at the boxed stuff again. It's creamy, delicious, and good for you.

INGREDIENTS | SERVES 4

10 ounces cream cheese, softened

⅓ cup heavy whipping cream

8 drops liquid stevia

1 tablespoon sugar-free pistachio syrup

½ cup crushed pistachios

Pop Some Pistachios

One-half cup of pistachios provides 5 percent of your copper needs for the entire day. Copper is an essential trace mineral that plays an important role in metabolism and the formation of red blood cells.

1. Beat cream cheese in a medium bowl until light and fluffy, about 2 minutes. Add whipping cream and beat until smooth.

2. Beat in stevia and pistachio syrup.

3. Stir in crushed pistachios.

4. Refrigerate until firm, about 45 minutes to 1 hour.

5. Serve chilled.

Mint Chocolate Chip Ice Cream

When you hear the words "ice cream," avocados may not be the first thing that comes to mind, but they give this recipe a rich, creamy texture and you won't even be able to taste them.

INGREDIENTS | SERVES 2

2 large ripe avocados

1 (13.5-ounce) can full-fat coconut milk

½ cup granulated erythritol

1 teaspoon vanilla extract

½ teaspoon peppermint extract

2 squares 90% dark chocolate

Mint leaves (optional)

No Ice-Cream Maker? No Worries!

Even if you don't have an ice-cream maker, you can still enjoy this ice cream. Pour the mixed ingredients in a stainless steel bowl and put in the freezer for about 20 minutes. Once the edges of the mixture start to freeze, whisk the mixture rapidly until smooth and creamy. Repeat this every 20–30 minutes until ice cream forms.

1. Cut avocados in half and scoop out flesh into a medium steel mixing bowl. Add coconut milk and beat until smooth. Add granulated erythritol, vanilla extract, and peppermint extract. Beat until smooth.

2. Grate chocolate with a handheld grater and fold shavings into cream mixture.

3. Pour liquid into an ice-cream maker, following manufacturer's instructions.

4. Garnish with mint leaves if desired. Serve frozen.

Chocolate Chip Cookies

Being on a ketogenic diet doesn't mean you have to miss out on classic chocolate chip cookies. This version rivals the real thing, but with none of the unhealthy refined sugar.

INGREDIENTS | SERVES 16

½ cup butter, softened
¼ cup granulated erythritol
1 teaspoon vanilla extract
2 large eggs
1 cup almond flour
⅓ cup coconut flour
1 teaspoon baking powder
¼ teaspoon salt
4 ounces unsweetened baking chocolate, chopped

1. Preheat oven to 350°F.

2. In a medium bowl, beat butter until light and fluffy, about 2 minutes. Beat in erythritol, vanilla, and eggs until smooth.

3. In a small bowl, combine almond flour, coconut flour, baking powder, and salt.

4. Fold flour mixture into egg mixture. Add chocolate chunks.

5. Drop by the tablespoonful onto a cookie sheet. Bake for 10 minutes.

Coconut Whipped Cream

Don't cut corners with this recipe. Making sure the coconut milk is fully chilled before whipping can make the difference between ending up with whipped cream or a sloppy mess.

INGREDIENTS | YIELDS 1½ CUPS

1 (13.5-ounce) can full-fat coconut milk
3 teaspoons powdered erythritol
½ teaspoon vanilla extract

Find the Right Milk

Unfortunately, there is a bit of inconsistency when it comes to canned coconut milk. Some brands whip up nicely while others seem to fall flat. If you've followed the directions closely and still can't get a nice whipped cream, try a different brand of coconut milk—and make sure it's full fat.

1. Refrigerate can of coconut milk for 24 hours.

2. Place small mixing bowl and beaters into freezer for 20 minutes.

3. Carefully remove the can of coconut milk from the refrigerator, making sure not to shake or tip it. Open can and use a spoon to scoop out the coconut cream that has risen to the top. Put coconut cream in chilled bowl.

4. Beat the coconut cream with a handheld beater until peaks begin to form, about 3 minutes.

5. Add in powdered erythritol and vanilla and beat until combined.

6. Serve immediately.

Walnut Blondies

These walnut blondies are divine warm with a scoop of ice cream or a dollop of Coconut Whipped Cream on top (see recipe in this chapter).

INGREDIENTS | SERVES 16

1 cup butter
1 cup granulated erythritol
1 large egg
1 teaspoon vanilla extract
⅛ teaspoon salt
1¼ cups almond flour
¾ cup crushed walnuts
2 squares 90% dark chocolate, crushed

1. Preheat oven to 350°F. Grease an 8" × 8" baking pan.

2. Melt butter in a medium microwave-safe mixing bowl. Add granulated erythritol and beat until smooth. Beat in egg and vanilla.

3. Stir in salt and almond flour. Fold in walnuts and dark chocolate pieces.

4. Bake for 20 minutes or until a toothpick inserted in the center comes out clean.

Pumpkin Donut Holes

These donut holes are the perfect bite-sized treat, especially around the holidays. Just make sure to use pure pumpkin purée instead of premade pumpkin pie filling, which is loaded with sugar.

INGREDIENTS | SERVES 24

2 cups almond flour
¼ cup granulated erythritol
½ teaspoon salt
1 teaspoon baking soda
1 tablespoon pumpkin pie seasoning
2 large eggs
¾ cup canned pumpkin purée
¼ cup butter, melted
2 tablespoons cream cheese
1 teaspoon vanilla extract
¼ teaspoon maple extract

1. Preheat oven to 325°F.

2. Grease the wells of a 24-cup mini muffin tin.

3. Combine almond flour, erythritol, salt, baking soda, and pumpkin pie seasoning in a medium bowl. Stir until combined.

4. In a small bowl, beat eggs, pumpkin, melted butter, cream cheese, vanilla extract, and maple extract until smooth. Fold egg mixture into dry ingredients until just combined.

5. Drop by teaspoonfuls into each well of a mini muffin tin. Bake for 15 minutes or until a toothpick inserted in the center comes out clean.

6. Store at room temperature.

CHAPTER 15

Fat Bombs

Cocoa Coconut Butter Fat Bombs

In addition to coconut oil, this recipe uses coconut butter, which differs from the oil. Coconut butter is the puréed meat of mature coconuts, while coconut oil has been separated from the coconut meat. One cannot be substituted for the other.

INGREDIENTS | SERVES 12

1 cup coconut oil

½ cup butter

6 tablespoons unsweetened cocoa powder

15 drops liquid stevia

½ cup coconut butter

Make Your Own

Coconut butter isn't always easy to find. It's simple, and more cost effective, to make your own. To make 2 cups of coconut butter, put 6 cups of unsweetened coconut flakes into a blender with a pinch of salt and blend until completely smooth. This usually takes 5–6 minutes.

1. Put coconut oil, butter, unsweetened cocoa powder, and stevia in a small saucepan, stirring frequently until all ingredients are melted.

2. Melt coconut butter in a separate small pan.

3. Pour 2 tablespoons of cocoa mixture into each well of a 12-cup silicone mold.

4. Add 1 tablespoon of melted coconut butter to each well.

5. Place in the freezer until hardened, about 30 minutes.

6. Store in the refrigerator.

Almond Butter Fat Bombs

You can replace the almond butter in this recipe with any nut butter of your choice. Cashew butter and peanut butter work really well, too. Just make sure that your nut butter doesn't contain any added sugar.

INGREDIENTS | SERVES 12

⅓ cup coconut oil

⅓ cup butter

⅓ cup unsweetened almond butter

2 tablespoons cream cheese

15 drops liquid stevia

Do It Yourself!

Making your own almond butter is simple and a great way to ensure that it doesn't contain any hidden sugar. Simply put almonds in a food processor and process until the oils break down and a nut butter forms. To up the fat content and make the almond butter smoother, add a couple of teaspoons of almond oil (or another oil of your choice).

1. Place all ingredients in a small saucepan and stir over medium-low heat until all ingredients are melted and mixed together.

2. Pour an equal amount of mixture into each well of a 12-cup silicone mold.

3. Place in the freezer until hardened, about 30 minutes.

4. Store in the refrigerator.

Raspberry Cheesecake Fat Bombs

You can replace the raspberries in this recipe with blackberries, blueberries, or strawberries. Combine them all for a delicious mixed berry cheesecake bomb.

INGREDIENTS | SERVES 12

½ cup frozen raspberries

10 drops liquid stevia

1 teaspoon vanilla extract

¾ cup cream cheese, room temperature

¼ cup coconut oil, room temperature

Be Careful with Berries

Berries are full of fiber so their net carbohydrate count is not as high as some other fruits. In fact, 1 cup contains 7 net carbohydrates. You still need to be careful when eating berries on a ketogenic diet. Don't overdo it and always make sure to count your macronutrients to make sure that berries fit into your plan that day.

1. Place raspberries in a food processer and process until smooth. Add stevia and vanilla extract and process until incorporated.

2. Add cream cheese and coconut oil and process until all ingredients are well combined.

3. Place an equal amount of mixture in each well of a 12-cup silicone mold.

4. Place in freezer until hardened, about 30 minutes.

5. Store in the refrigerator.

Cashew Butter Cup Fat Bombs

Many commercially available cashew butters contain an added sweetener, so be careful when choosing one. If you can't find one at the store, you can always make your own.

INGREDIENTS | SERVES 12

1 cup coconut oil

¾ cup butter, divided

6 tablespoons unsweetened cocoa powder

15 drops liquid stevia

¼ cup sugar-free cashew butter

2 tablespoons heavy whipping cream

Nut Butters at Home

Making cashew butter is the same basic process as making coconut butter. To make about 1½ cups of cashew butter, put 2 cups of unroasted, unsalted cashews in a food processor with a pinch of salt and 1 tablespoon of coconut oil. Process for about 30 seconds and then scrape down the sides of the food processor. Continue processing until smooth, scraping the sides when necessary. Be patient, as the process can take several minutes.

1. Put coconut oil, ½ cup of the butter, cocoa powder, and stevia in a small saucepan and stir over medium heat until melted and well combined.

2. Pour an equal amount of the mixture into each well of a mini muffin tin lined with cupcake wrappers. Place muffin tin in the freezer and allow to harden, about 30 minutes.

3. Place remaining ¼ cup butter, cashew butter, and whipping cream in a small bowl and beat with a hand-held mixer until combined and fluffy.

4. Once the chocolate mixture in the freezer has hardened, spoon an equal amount of the cashew butter mixture on top of each well and place in the freezer. Allow to harden, at least 30 minutes.

5. Store in refrigerator.

Coconut Peppermint Fat Bombs

You can replace the peppermint extract in this recipe with any other pure extract. Try lemon, orange, almond, or maple.

INGREDIENTS | SERVES 12

1 cup coconut butter
¼ cup unsweetened shredded coconut
1 tablespoon coconut oil
½ teaspoon peppermint extract

1. Put all ingredients in a small saucepan and heat over low heat until melted and well combined.

2. Pour an equal amount of mixture into each well of a 12-cup muffin tin lined with cupcake wrappers.

3. Place in the freezer and allow to harden, about 30 minutes.

4. Store in the refrigerator.

Lemon Cheesecake Fat Bombs

Fresh lemon juice straight from the lemon is best for this recipe, but if you're out of lemons, you can use bottled versions, too.

INGREDIENTS | SERVES 12

¼ cup cream cheese, softened
⅔ cup butter
2 tablespoons heavy whipping cream
1 tablespoon lemon juice
¼ teaspoon lemon extract
10 drops liquid stevia

1. Beat cream cheese, butter, and whipping cream together in a small bowl until smooth. Add lemon juice, lemon extract, and stevia until combined.

2. Drop by tablespoons onto a cookie sheet lined with wax paper and place in the freezer until hardened, about 30 minutes.

3. Store in the refrigerator.

Cinnamon Bun Fat Bombs

These cinnamon bun fat bombs have the same flavor as a cinnamon roll fresh from the oven but without the sugar and carbohydrates.

INGREDIENTS | SERVES 12

1 cup coconut butter, softened

¼ teaspoon plus ⅛ teaspoon ground cinnamon

¼ teaspoon ground nutmeg

¼ teaspoon vanilla extract

¼ cup crushed walnuts

Smooth It Out

The crushed walnuts finish off these fat bombs with a nice crunch, but you could also grind the walnuts instead for a smooth, but still decadent, finish.

1. Combine coconut butter, ¼ teaspoon cinnamon, nutmeg, and vanilla extract in a small bowl and mix until well combined.

2. Separate the mixture into 12 equal parts and roll into ball shapes. Place on a cookie sheet lined with wax paper.

3. Mix crushed walnuts with remaining cinnamon in a small bowl. Roll balls in nut mixture until coated.

4. Place finished balls on a cookie sheet lined with wax paper and refrigerate until ready to eat.

5. Store in the refrigerator.

Mixed Nut Butter Bombs

The combination of cashew butter, peanut flour,
and almond extract is enough to satisfy every nut lover's craving.

INGREDIENTS | SERVES 12

½ cup cashew butter

1 cup defatted unsweetened peanut flour

¼ cup butter, melted

¼ teaspoon almond extract

Defatting Peanuts

Defatted peanut flour is a peanut flour that has had a large percentage of its fat removed through a mechanical process. The fat content of defatted peanut flour still falls around 25 percent of calories, but the shelf life is significantly increased.

1. Mix cashew butter and peanut flour together in a small bowl until well combined.

2. Stir in melted butter until smooth. Add almond extract and stir until combined.

3. Scoop out tablespoons of mixture onto a cookie sheet covered in wax paper.

4. Place in the freezer until hardened, about 30 minutes.

5. Store in the refrigerator.

Peanut Butter Fat Bombs

The crunchy peanut butter and crushed peanuts in this recipe give these peanut butter fat bombs an unbeatable texture. If you prefer less crunch, use smooth peanut butter instead.

INGREDIENTS | SERVES 12

1 cup coconut oil
½ cup butter
½ cup crunchy peanut butter
2 tablespoons cream cheese
10 drops liquid stevia
¼ cup crushed unsalted peanuts

1. Place coconut oil, butter, peanut butter, cream cheese, and stevia in a small saucepan and stir over medium heat until melted.

2. Sprinkle crushed peanuts evenly in each well of a 12-cup mini muffin pan. Pour peanut butter mixture over the peanuts.

3. Place in the freezer until hardened, about 30 minutes.

4. Store in the refrigerator.

Maple Fat Bombs

*These Maple Fat Bombs provide comforting maple flavor
without all of the carbohydrates contained in regular maple syrup.*

INGREDIENTS | SERVES 12

¼ cup butter

½ cup coconut butter

10 drops liquid stevia

½ teaspoon maple extract

¼ teaspoon ground cinnamon

½ cup crushed walnuts

Choosing Your Maple

There are four different types of maple extract: pure, natural, imitation, and artificial. Imitation and artificial extracts are made in a lab and often contain no real maple product at all. Stick to pure or natural extracts.

1. Place butter, coconut butter, stevia, maple extract, and cinnamon in a small saucepan and stir over medium heat until melted. Mix thoroughly.

2. Remove mixture from heat and stir in crushed walnuts.

3. Fill each well of a 12-cup mini muffin pan lined with cupcake wrappers or a silicone mold with an equal amount of the mixture.

4. Place pan or mold in the freezer until mixture hardens, about 30 minutes.

5. Store in the refrigerator.

Blueberry Fat Bombs

Blueberries and cream cheese are a winning combination, but if you want a different flavor, make this a triple berry fat bomb by using a combination of blueberries, blackberries, and strawberries.

INGREDIENTS | SERVES 12

¾ cup blueberries, divided

¼ cup coconut cream

⅓ cup cream cheese, softened

½ cup coconut butter, melted

½ cup coconut oil, melted

8 drops liquid stevia

Use What You've Got

Silicone molds are extremely helpful when you're on a ketogenic diet, especially if you're planning to make fat bombs a regular part of your diet. If you don't want to purchase silicone molds, you can use ice cube trays, but it will be harder to remove the bombs from the tray.

1. Place ½ cup of the berries, coconut cream, and cream cheese in a food processor and process until smooth. Add melted coconut butter, melted coconut oil, and liquid stevia and process again until smooth.

2. Fill up each well of a 12-cup silicone mold or mini muffin tin lined with cupcake wrappers with an equal amount of the blueberry mixture and drop the remaining blueberries on top.

3. Place in the freezer until hardened, about 30 minutes. Store in the refrigerator.

Chocolate Orange Fat Bombs

The citrus notes in the orange extract in this recipe bring out the flavor of the unsweetened cocoa powder. You can make this a double-chocolate fat bomb instead by swapping out the orange extract for chocolate extract.

INGREDIENTS | SERVES 12

½ cup butter

½ cup coconut oil

5 tablespoons unsweetened cocoa powder

1 teaspoon orange extract

1. Mix all ingredients together in a small saucepan over medium-low heat until melted and smooth.

2. Pour into each well of a 12-cup silicone mold and place into the freezer until hardened, about 30 minutes.

3. Store in the refrigerator.

Vanilla Macadamia Fat Bombs

You can skip the first step in this recipe by purchasing macadamia nut flour instead of grinding whole macadamia nuts, but it can be more expensive that way.

INGREDIENTS | SERVES 12

½ cup macadamia nuts

1 cup cream cheese, softened

½ cup heavy whipping cream

1 teaspoon vanilla extract

⅛ teaspoon salt

10 drops liquid stevia

1. Place macadamia nuts in a food processor and process until you achieve a fine meal consistency. Add remaining ingredients and process until smooth.

2. Pour mixture into each well of a 12-cup silicone mold and freeze until hardened, about 30 minutes.

3. Store in the refrigerator.

Macadamia Knowledge

There are an estimated seven species of macadamia nuts around the world, but only two species are edible. The majority of macadamia nuts come from Australia, but the nuts that come from Hawaii are often described as the best-tasting.

Pumpkin Fat Bombs

For a richer taste, swap out the coconut oil in this recipe for unsalted butter. Keep the amount of coconut butter the same.

INGREDIENTS | SERVES 12

½ cup coconut butter, softened

¼ cup coconut oil, softened

⅛ cup pumpkin purée

1 teaspoon pumpkin pie spice

¼ teaspoon vanilla extract

8 drops liquid stevia

⅛ teaspoon salt

Go for the Gourd

Canned pumpkin is about 90 percent water, so it contains very few calories—fewer than 50 per serving. Pumpkin is also rich in fiber, containing 7 grams per cup, but it's not considered a low-carbohydrate food. Pumpkin can be incorporated into a ketogenic diet, but always watch your portions.

1. Mix all ingredients together in a small bowl and stir until combined.

2. Pour into an 8" × 8" baking pan and spread out mixture evenly. Refrigerate for 30 minutes and then cut into 12 squares.

Avocado Fat Bomb Smoothie

The avocado in this recipe will make your smoothie nice and creamy without changing the flavor.

INGREDIENTS | SERVES 2

1 cup full-fat coconut milk

½ large avocado

¼ cup ice

1 teaspoon vanilla extract

1 tablespoon granulated erythritol

2 tablespoons coconut butter

Combine all ingredients in blender and blend until smooth. Serve immediately.

CHAPTER 16

Smoothies

Coconut Chia Smoothie

You can turn this into a chocolate coconut chia smoothie by adding a couple of tablespoons of unsweetened cocoa powder before blending.

INGREDIENTS | SERVES 1

1 cup full-fat canned coconut milk
2 tablespoons chia seeds
2 tablespoons coconut oil, melted
¼ cup frozen blueberries

1. Place all ingredients in a blender and blend until smooth.

2. Serve cold.

Choosing Coconut Milk

The coconut milk that comes in a box is full of preservatives and low in fat. Some sweetened varieties contain sugar or other sweeteners that increase carbohydrate content. Look for full-fat coconut milk in a can that contains only coconut milk or a combination of coconut milk and guar gum.

Chocolate Almond Smoothie

Turn this into a chocolate coconut smoothie by using coconut milk and coconut butter instead of almond milk and almond butter.

INGREDIENTS | SERVES 2

1 cup unsweetened almond milk

¼ cup sugar-free almond butter

2 tablespoons unsweetened cocoa powder

¼ cup heavy cream

1½ cups ice

5 drops liquid stevia (optional)

1. Put all ingredients in a blender and blend until smooth.

2. Serve cold.

The Power of Stevia

Stevia contains no carbohydrates or calories, but is 200 times sweeter than sugar, so a little goes a long way. You can also use powdered stevia in place of liquid stevia, but the liquid versions tend to blend better, especially with cold liquids.

Pumpkin Pie Smoothie

Don't confuse pumpkin purée with canned pumpkin pie filling. Pure pumpkin purée contains only the flesh of a pumpkin, while pumpkin pie filling contains sweeteners that increase sugar and carbohydrate content.

INGREDIENTS | SERVES 2

½ cup pumpkin purée

1 cup full-fat canned coconut milk

½ teaspoon pumpkin pie spice

¼ large avocado

2 tablespoons coconut oil, melted

¼ teaspoon maple extract

¼ cup unsweetened whey protein powder

1. Put all ingredients in a blender and blend until smooth.

2. Serve cold.

Green Smoothie

The type of whey protein powder you choose for this recipe will make a big difference in the taste. Switch it up by alternating between chocolate and vanilla.

INGREDIENTS | SERVES 2

1 cup full-fat canned coconut milk
½ avocado
¼ cup whey protein powder
½ teaspoon vanilla extract
½ cup baby spinach
2 drops liquid stevia

1. Put all ingredients in a blender and blend until smooth.

2. Serve immediately.

Watch Your Whey

Although protein is the major nutrient in protein powders, a lot of them contain sweeteners that add a significant amount of carbohydrates. When choosing a protein powder, look for one that is low in net carbohydrates and doesn't contain artificial ingredients.

Honeydew and Avocado Smoothie

This creamy, sweet smoothie packs plenty of protein and healthy fats to keep you full and going strong throughout the day. Try substituting cantaloupe or your favorite melon for a slightly different flavor.

INGREDIENTS | SERVES 1

¼ medium avocado, peeled and pit removed

¼ cup chunks honeydew melon

½ cup full-fat canned coconut milk

¼ cup water

1 tablespoon chia seeds

2 tablespoons unsweetened whey protein powder

Ice, to thicken, if desired

1. Place avocado, melon, coconut milk, water, chia seeds, and protein powder in a blender and blend until smooth.

2. Add ice to thicken, if desired.

3. Serve cold.

Honeydew and Cantaloupe: Sweet Treats

Honeydew melon is related to the cantaloupe, but it has a smooth green flesh and a slightly milder flavor. Both fruits are often served for dessert. You can consume more than half of the recommended daily amount of vitamin C with just one wedge of honeydew melon; one wedge of cantaloupe will provide over 100 percent of the recommended daily amount of vitamin C, and 120 percent of vitamin A.

Carrot Asparagus Green Smoothie

The addition of flaxseed to this smoothie lends a delicious hint of nutty flavor, and boosts the vitamin and mineral content as well.

INGREDIENTS | SERVES 4

1 cup watercress

1 cup chopped asparagus

2 small carrots, peeled and chopped

2 tablespoons flaxseed

2 cups full-fat canned coconut milk

1 cup water

1. Combine watercress, asparagus, carrots, flaxseed, and coconut milk in a blender and blend until thoroughly combined.

2. Add water while blending until desired texture is reached.

Flaxseed

Flaxseed is a common product found in almost every grocery store. Available organic, nonorganic, ground, and whole, flaxseed can be found in aisles with nuts or near produce. You can purchase the whole seed product and use them in sandwiches, salads, and main dishes by using a coffee grinder and grinding them until thoroughly powdered.

Avocado Raspberry Smoothie

Sweet and satisfying, this smoothie makes a great breakfast—or a decadent dessert. Try swapping out the raspberries with blueberries, blackberries, or even cloudberries for a more exotic touch.

INGREDIENTS | SERVES 1

¼ medium avocado, peeled and pit removed

¼ cup raspberries

½ cup chopped fresh mint

1 cup heavy cream

2 tablespoons coconut oil, melted

½ cup water

1. Place avocado, raspberries, mint, cream, and coconut oil in a blender and blend until smooth.

2. Add water while blending until desired consistency is reached.

Arctic Cloudberries

Tiny golden cloudberries are one of nature's gifts in Scandinavia's harshly beautiful mountains, as much the hallmark of the culinary *terroir* as grapes are to Italy's far gentler climes. You're unlikely to find cloudberries fresh in most parts of the United States, although they do grow wild across northern Canada, where they're called bakeapples. Some IKEA stores sell frozen cloudberries, as well as cloudberry jam—but be wary of the jam's high amounts of sugar and carbohydrates.

Lime and Coconut Smoothie

The tart taste of lime in this green smoothie is balanced with the sweet and creamy coconut milk. This recipe will bring the tastes of tropical locales into your kitchen, and is great to share with friends.

INGREDIENTS | SERVES 4

1 cup fresh spinach
2 tablespoons chia seeds
2 large limes, peeled and seeded
2 cups full-fat canned coconut milk
½ cup purified water

1. Combine spinach, chia seeds, limes, and coconut milk in a blender with half of the water and blend until thoroughly combined.

2. Add remaining water while blending until desired consistency is reached.

Limes and Joints

Although many patients suffering from arthritis decide to exercise and eat differently, few know the powerful effects limes can have on joints! These vitamin C–filled fruits can pack a punch in reducing arthritis symptoms to a minimum and making everyday life seem less achy!

Triple Green Smoothie

This smoothie features spinach, avocado, and lime for a boost of vitamins, whole nutrition, and a balance of flavors. If the taste of spinach is too strong for your palate, try substituting romaine lettuce or watercress.

INGREDIENTS | SERVES 4

1 cup fresh spinach
2 avocados, peeled and pits removed
1 large lime, peeled and seeded
1 cup full-fat coconut milk, divided
¾ cup full-fat plain Greek yogurt, divided

1. Combine spinach, avocados, lime, ½ cup coconut milk, and ½ cup yogurt in a blender and blend until thoroughly combined.

2. Add remaining ½ cup coconut milk and ½ cup yogurt while blending until desired texture is reached.

Fiber Benefits

Leafy greens, vegetables, and fruits all contain some amount of this miracle substance. Because the human body is almost completely unable to digest fiber, we benefit from its tendency to make our stomachs feel full and clear our intestinal tracts by remaining nearly intact throughout digestion. Although fiber is available in pill and powder forms, those are a far cry from a healthy bowl of spinach or broccoli.

Ginger Strawberry Smoothie

The soothing effects of ginger make this recipe perfect for optimizing digestion. If you prefer a thicker, colder shake, add crushed ice ½ cup at a time until suitably thick and creamy.

INGREDIENTS | SERVES 4

1 cup watercress

¾ cup frozen strawberries

½" piece gingerroot, peeled

1 cup full-fat canned coconut milk

1 cup heavy cream, divided

1. Combine watercress, strawberries, ginger, coconut milk, and ½ cup heavy cream in a blender and blend until thoroughly combined.

2. Add remaining heavy cream as needed while blending until desired consistency is reached.

Almond Berry Smoothie

Almonds are the star of this flavorful smoothie—almond butter and whole almonds combine for a mix of crunchy and smooth textures. The omega-3 content of this smoothie is boosted with the addition of flaxseed, which adds even nuttier flavor.

INGREDIENTS | SERVES 4

2 cups unsweetened homemade almond milk, divided (see sidebar in Banana Nut Smoothie recipe)

2 tablespoons unsweetened almond butter

¼ cup raw almonds

1 tablespoon flaxseed

1 cup fresh spinach

1 cup strawberries

½ cup heavy cream

1. Combine 1 cup almond milk with the almond butter, almonds, and flaxseed in a blender and emulsify. For a smoother texture, emulsify completely until no nut pieces remain. For a chunky texture, be sure to leave some pieces of almond intact.

2. Add spinach, strawberries, and heavy cream and blend until thoroughly combined.

3. Add remaining 1 cup of almond milk as needed while blending until desired consistency is reached.

Strawberries for Sight

Rich in the antioxidants that give them their vibrant red color, this sweet berry is also rich in vitamins A, C, D, and E, B vitamins, folate, and phytochemicals that join forces to help you maintain healthy eyes and strong vision. Strawberries may help delay the onset of macular degeneration.

Kale and Brazil Nut Smoothie

This unusual blend of ingredients delivers sound nutrition and unique flavor. Kale is a nutritional powerhouse that provides an abundance of vitamins A and K. Ninety-one percent of Brazil nuts' calories come from fat, making them a perfect addition to the ketogenic diet.

INGREDIENTS | SERVES 2

2 cups chopped kale

¼ cup Brazil nuts, frozen

2 tablespoons coconut oil, melted

2 cups full-fat canned coconut milk

½ teaspoon ground cinnamon

½ teaspoon ground allspice

½–1 cup ice, as needed

1. Place kale, nuts, coconut oil, coconut milk, cinnamon, and allspice in a blender and blend until thoroughly combined.

2. With the blender running, add ice in small batches until desired consistency is reached. If smoothie is too thick, add splashes of water to thin out the consistency.

Brazil Nut Ecology

Brazil nuts grow on large, old-growth trees in the Amazon. These trees can live to be 500 years old, and their pollination (and nut production) depends on the presence of a particular species of orchid that attracts a particular bee. Brazil nuts are one of the Amazon's potential sustainable resources because they can be harvested each year without damaging the trees, but the nut production requires a delicate environmental balance that is being threatened by deforestation.

Calming Cucumber Smoothie

The light taste of cucumber and the refreshing fragrance of mint combine with romaine lettuce in this delightful smoothie. Toasted almonds make a great addition to this smoothie; try adding a tablespoon of sliced toasted almonds in addition to the coconut flakes.

INGREDIENTS | SERVES 4

1 cup chopped romaine lettuce

2 cucumbers, peeled

¼ cup chopped mint

1 cup full-fat canned coconut milk, divided

¼ cup unsweetened coconut flakes

1. Combine romaine, cucumbers, mint, and ½ cup coconut milk in a blender and combine thoroughly.

2. Add remaining coconut milk while blending.

3. Divide smoothie mixture into 4 glasses. Top each glass with 1 tablespoon coconut flakes to garnish.

Cucumbers Aren't Just Water

Even though a cucumber is mostly water (and fiber), it is far more than a tasty, thirst-quenching, and filling snack option. These green veggies have detoxifying and rehydrating properties. By consuming one serving of cucumbers per day, you'll not only fulfill a full serving of veggies and stave off hunger, you'll have clear, hydrated skin!

Spiced Cashew Butter Smoothie

Mix up the usual peanut butter– and almond butter–filled smoothies by swapping in cashew butter instead! Cashew butter is slightly sweet and very creamy. Raw cashew butter is best, as it contains higher levels of nutrients than its roasted counterparts.

INGREDIENTS | SERVES 1

½ avocado, peeled and pit removed

1 tablespoon unsweetened cashew butter

½ cup heavy cream

½ cup full-fat canned coconut milk

½ teaspoon ground cinnamon

½ teaspoon ground allspice

½ teaspoon sugar-free vanilla extract

½ cup ice

1 teaspoon crushed cashews (optional)

1. Combine avocado, cashew butter, heavy cream, coconut milk, cinnamon, allspice, and vanilla extract in a blender and combine thoroughly.

2. Slowly add ice while blending until desired texture is reached.

3. Pour smoothie mixture into a glass and top with 1 teaspoon crushed cashews, if desired.

Cashew Benefits

Cashews have a lower fat content than most nuts, but that does not mean they're not a great addition to the ketogenic diet. Cashews are high in heart-healthy monounsaturated fats, such as those found in olive oil, and have been found to reduce high triglycerides in the blood. In general, nuts promote heart health and lower the risk of weight gain, so add more servings to your diet to live your best!

Spiced Chocolate Smoothie

The flavors in this smoothie are reminiscent of Mexican hot chocolate—without all the added sugar and carbohydrates the traditional version contains. If cayenne powder is too spicy for your taste buds, simply omit it from this smoothie. Try adding a pinch of nutmeg instead.

INGREDIENTS | SERVES 1

½ cup full-fat canned coconut milk

1 tablespoon coconut oil, melted

1 tablespoon ground flaxseed or chia seeds

¼ teaspoon cayenne powder

½ teaspoon ground cinnamon

2½ tablespoons unsweetened cocoa powder

¼ teaspoon unsweetened vanilla extract

½ cup water

½ cup ice, if desired

1 cinnamon stick, to garnish

1. Combine coconut milk, coconut oil, ground seeds, cayenne, cinnamon, cocoa powder, vanilla extract, and water in a blender and combine thoroughly.

2. Slowly add ice while blending until desired texture is reached.

3. Pour smoothie mixture into a glass and garnish with cinnamon stick, if desired.

Cayenne for Digestive Health

You would think that such a spicy addition would cause stomach discomfort, but this pepper has amazing benefits. Cayenne has the ability to promote a digestive enzyme that works to kill bad bacteria ingested from foods while promoting the good bacteria that optimizes the digestive process. Cayenne also fights off the bad bacteria that cause stomach ulcers!

Coconut Cream Dream Smoothie

Coconut cream pie is a delicious dessert, but it packs empty calories and very few vitamins and minerals. This recipe blends the star ingredients of coconut cream pie in a healthy green smoothie.

INGREDIENTS | SERVES 4

1 cup chopped romaine lettuce

Flesh of 2 mature coconuts

1 tablespoon lemon juice

1 medium avocado, peeled and pit removed

¼" piece gingerroot, peeled

½ cup full-fat canned coconut milk

½ cup full-fat plain Greek-style yogurt

1 cup ice (or to taste)

1. Combine romaine, coconut flesh, lemon juice, avocado, ginger, and coconut milk in a blender until thoroughly combined.

2. Add the yogurt while blending until just combined.

3. Slowly add ice while blending until desired texture is reached.

Orange Coconut Smoothie

Packed with brain-stimulating and immune-system-boosting vitamin C, this smoothie is a great option when everyone around you seems to be sick. Its power is intensified with the antioxidant-rich coconut milk.

INGREDIENTS | SERVES 4

1 cup chopped iceberg lettuce

2 medium oranges, peeled

2 cups full-fat canned coconut milk

2 tablespoons coconut oil, melted

1. Blend lettuce and oranges until just combined.

2. Add coconut milk and coconut oil slowly while blending until desired consistency is reached.

Vitamin C

Oranges are well known for their immunity-building power, and rightfully so! Consuming oranges every day can help the human body can fight off illnesses from the common cold to serious cancers and heart disease. You can thank the rich beta-carotenes and the vitamin C. An orange is a definite must for health and longevity.

Banana Nut Smoothie

This smoothie combines ample protein and the healthy fats you need. In addition to the vitamins, minerals, and nutrients from the lettuce and banana, the healthy fats from the coconut milk make this smoothie a powerful start to any day.

INGREDIENTS | SERVES 4

1 cup full-fat canned coconut milk

1 cup chopped iceberg lettuce

1 cup heavy cream

½ teaspoon vanilla extract

1 cup homemade unsweetened vanilla almond milk

1 medium banana, sliced

1. Combine coconut milk, lettuce, heavy cream, and vanilla extract in a blender with ½ cup almond milk and blend thoroughly.

2. Continue adding remaining almond milk while blending until desired consistency is reached.

3. To serve, divide smoothie into 4 glasses. Top each glass with an equal amount of sliced banana.

Make Your Own Almond Milk

Although there are a number of almond milks on the market, they are often full of sugar or unhealthy additives. Some people choose to create their own lower-cost, lower-sugar version at home. If you'd like to create your own almond milk, combine ½ cup water and 1 cup almonds and blend thoroughly. Add a touch of vanilla extract to make a vanilla version. Strain before using.

Slow Cooker Recipes

Meaty Chili

This recipe calls for a mixture of bacon and pork, but you can use any combination of ground meat that you want.

INGREDIENTS | SERVES 8

8 slices thick-cut sugar-free bacon

1 medium white onion, chopped

1 large green pepper, diced

1 small red pepper, diced

1 pound ground beef

1 pound ground pork

1 (14.5-ounce) can fire-roasted diced tomatoes

1 (6-ounce) can tomato paste

3 tablespoons chili powder

1 tablespoon cumin

1 teaspoon garlic powder

2 teaspoons sugar-free hot sauce

1 teaspoon salt

1 cup sugar-free beef broth

1. Cook bacon over medium-high heat in a large skillet until crisp, about 10 minutes.

2. Remove bacon from heat, reserving bacon fat, and chop into small pieces.

3. Put chopped onions and peppers in the same skillet in hot bacon grease and sauté until translucent, 3–4 minutes. Add ground beef and ground pork and cook until no longer pink. Drain liquid.

4. Put beef mixture, chopped bacon, and remaining ingredients in a slow cooker. Stir until ingredients are combined and cook on low for 6 hours.

Searching for Sugar

Not all hot sauces are the same. Some of them contain sugar, even though it's not necessary. Check your hot sauce labels and choose one that is sugar-free. A lot of popular brands fall into this category.

Classic Sloppy Joes

This traditional sandwich filling makes a great keto recipe to stuff into peppers, spoon over roasted spaghetti squash, or use as a dip for sliced vegetables. It also makes a great party dish. Make ahead at your convenience, then chill or freeze. Reheat in your slow cooker just before your party.

INGREDIENTS | SERVES 8

4 tablespoons olive oil

2 onions, peeled and thinly sliced

1 clove garlic, minced

1 pound 85/15 ground beef

1 pound ground pork

½ cup apple cider vinegar

½ cup tomato paste

¼ teaspoon salt

½ teaspoon black pepper

1. Heat the oil in a large skillet over low heat. Sauté the onions in the skillet over low heat until soft, about 12–15 minutes. For the last 2 minutes of cooking, add the garlic. Stir until cooked and fragrant. Transfer to the slow cooker.

2. Brown the meat in the same pan over medium heat, breaking into chunks; drain. Add the meat, vinegar, tomato paste, salt, and pepper to the slow cooker.

3. Cover and heat on a low setting for 3–4 hours.

Quick Tomato Peeling

Not everyone likes peeled tomatoes. Sometimes the presence of the peels adds just a bit more color and texture. But if you do peel, there is a helpful trick. Arrange the tomatoes in a bowl. Cover them with boiling water for 2 minutes, then drain. This will loosen the skins for easier peeling.

Beef Stew

This dish is great to come home to on a cold wintry night. It's very simple, and you can set it to cook and leave it alone until it's done.

INGREDIENTS | SERVES 6

1 tablespoon coconut oil

2 pounds stew meat

1 green pepper, coarsely chopped

3 cups pearl onions, peeled

30 cherry tomatoes

1 tablespoon tapioca flour

2 tablespoons granulated erythritol

½ teaspoon salt

¼ teaspoon black pepper

1. Heat the coconut oil in a large skillet over medium heat. Sauté the meat in oil until browned on all sides, then drain and transfer meat to the slow cooker.

2. Place the green pepper, onions, tomatoes, tapioca flour, granulated erythritol, salt, and pepper in the slow cooker.

3. Cover and heat on a low setting for 4–5 hours.

Ginger Barbecue Beef

Fresh ginger has a much more potent flavor than powdered, dried ginger. Try to use the fresh root if available.

INGREDIENTS | SERVES 6–8

3 cloves garlic, peeled and minced

1" fresh gingerroot, peeled and minced

½ cup coconut aminos

½ cup water

2 tablespoons sesame oil

2 tablespoons granulated erythritol

4 teaspoons sesame seeds

3 pounds beef

1 onion

1. Mix garlic and gingerroot in a small bowl with coconut aminos, water, oil, erythritol, and sesame seeds.

2. Cut the beef in slices. Peel and coarsely chop the onion.

3. Arrange the beef and onion in the slow cooker. Pour the sauce mixture over the beef and onions, making sure they are completely coated.

4. Cover and heat on a low setting for 4–5 hours.

Coconut Soup

This simple dish is deliciously smooth and creamy. You can add cooked beef, chicken, or seafood for other flavors and textures.

INGREDIENTS | SERVES 6–8

3 tablespoons butter
1 medium onion, finely chopped
1½ tablespoons tapioca flour
5 cups sugar-free chicken broth, divided
2 cups unsweetened coconut flakes
1¼ cups full-fat canned coconut milk
¼ cup chopped fresh cilantro, optional

1. Melt the butter in a large skillet over medium heat. Sauté the onion in butter until soft, about 10 minutes.

2. Blend the tapioca flour into ½ cup of the chicken broth. Add to the onion and stir over medium heat until thickened.

3. Transfer the mixture to the slow cooker and add the remaining broth.

4. Cover and heat on a low setting for 2–3 hours.

5. Preheat the oven to 350°F. Place the coconut flakes in a single layer on a baking sheet. Toast in the oven for 10 minutes, stirring occasionally, until the coconut is slightly browned.

6. An hour before serving, add the coconut milk to the slow cooker. Stir to combine.

7. To serve, ladle the soup into bowls and sprinkle with toasted coconut. Alternatively, you can add the cooked meat of your choice, and sprinkle with freshly chopped cilantro.

Country Chicken Stew

This recipe takes some advance planning, but it's a sure way to impress dinner guests. Serve this with sliced avocado and plenty of sour cream.

INGREDIENTS | SERVES 4–6

2 pounds chicken thighs, cut into pieces

1 large carrot, peeled and chopped

1 large onion, peeled and chopped

1 cup sugar-free chicken stock

2 cups water, divided

1 bouquet garni

1 teaspoon whole black peppercorns

2 tablespoons butter, divided

1 tablespoon tapioca flour

¼ pound salt pork

10 pearl onions

½ pound mushrooms

1 tablespoon fresh chopped parsley

Too Salty?

If your soup is too salty, put a piece of raw potato in the soup or add a spoonful each of cider vinegar and erythritol. If soup is too greasy, drop in a lettuce leaf, then take it back out after 2 minutes. The leaf will take some grease along with it.

1. Place the chicken thighs, carrot, onion, stock, 1 cup water, bouquet garni, and peppercorns in a large zip-top plastic bag. Make sure the chicken is completely submerged in the marinade with the vegetables. Place in the refrigerator to marinate overnight.

2. After marinating overnight, remove the chicken; strain the marinade and save the juice, discarding the vegetables and spices.

3. Melt 1 tablespoon butter in a large skillet over medium heat and mix in the tapioca flour until blended. Add the marinated chicken, stir for a few minutes, then slowly stir in the strained marinade and the remaining 1 cup of water. Mix to make sure there are no lumps.

4. Transfer to the slow cooker. Cover and heat on a low setting for 4–6 hours.

5. Cube the salt pork and peel the pearl onions. Place the pork with the onions in a medium pot, and cover with water. Heat over high heat until boiling; drain and discard the liquid.

6. Clean the mushrooms by wiping with a damp cloth, then halve them. Sauté the boiled pork, boiled onions, and mushrooms in remaining butter in a large skillet over medium heat until the pork is browned. Drain, then transfer to the slow cooker with the meat.

7. Cover the slow cooker and heat on a low setting for another 2 hours. Before serving, stir in the parsley.

Venison Roast in Orange

If you don't have access to venison, substitute beef or pork. Use an inexpensive cut; the acidic orange juice will tenderize it during cooking.

INGREDIENTS | SERVES 8

3 pounds venison roast

2 slices sugar-free bacon, cut into small pieces

2 cloves garlic, minced

½ teaspoon salt

½ teaspoon black pepper

1 bay leaf

2 whole cloves

¼ cup orange juice

Don't Eat Bay Leaves

Remember, bay leaves add lots of flavor, but you should always remove them before serving a dish. Bay leaves are sharp and dangerous to eat.

1. In a large skillet, sauté the venison with the bacon, garlic, salt, and pepper over medium heat until the meat is lightly browned, about 5–8 minutes.

2. Transfer the meat and juices, bay leaf, cloves, and orange juice to the slow cooker.

3. Cover and heat on a low setting for 6–8 hours.

4. Open the slow cooker twice to baste, but no more. Remove the bay leaf before serving.

Pull-Apart Pork

This is excellent on keto "sandwiches," or served by itself. It also freezes well and can be stored in single-serving containers for quick meals.

INGREDIENTS | SERVES 6

1 tablespoon coconut oil
2 pounds pork stew meat, cubed
2 yellow onions, chopped
4 medium tomatoes, chopped
4 cloves garlic, minced
2 teaspoons hot chili powder
¼ teaspoon ground cinnamon
¼ teaspoon cayenne pepper
2 teaspoons dried oregano
2 teaspoons ground cumin
½ teaspoon salt
¼ cup apple cider vinegar

1. Melt the coconut oil in a large skillet over medium heat. Sauté the pork and onions in the oil until the meat is lightly browned, about 5–8 minutes.

2. Mix the tomatoes and garlic together in a large bowl.

3. Mix the spices, salt, and vinegar in a small bowl.

4. Place half of the tomato mixture in the bottom of the slow cooker. Sprinkle with ¼ of the spice mixture.

5. Place the meat mixture over the tomato layer, and sprinkle with ½ of the spice mixture.

6. Place the remaining tomato mixture on top of the meat, and sprinkle with the remaining spice mixture.

7. Cover and heat on a low setting for 6–8 hours.

Chicken Peanut Stew

Sprinkle with chopped peanuts and flaked coconut before serving over freshly cooked cauliflower "rice."

INGREDIENTS | SERVES 4

4 chicken breasts
1 large green bell pepper
2 medium yellow onions
1 (6-ounce) can tomato paste
¾ cup sugar-free crunchy peanut butter
3 cups sugar-free chicken broth
1 teaspoon salt
1 teaspoon chili powder
1 teaspoon granulated erythritol
½ teaspoon ground nutmeg

1. Remove the skin and bones from the chicken breasts and discard; cut the meat into 1" cubes.

2. Remove the stem and seeds from the pepper and cut into ¼" rings. Peel the onions and cut into ¼" rings.

3. Combine all the ingredients in the slow cooker; stir until all ingredients are well mingled.

4. Cover and cook on a low setting for 4–6 hours.

East Indian Green Curried Chicken

This incredible dish has complex flavors and a fiery heat. Serve over steamed cauliflower, Fried Cauliflower "Rice" (see recipe in Chapter 11), or Garlicky Green Beans (see recipe in Chapter 11).

INGREDIENTS | SERVES 6

6 chicken breasts

1½ cups unsweetened full-fat canned coconut milk, divided

1½ tablespoons green curry paste

½ cup sliced canned bamboo shoots

¼ cup fish sauce

1 tablespoon granulated erythritol

¼ cup chopped fresh mint leaves

2 fresh green chili peppers, minced

Stocking Up on Ethnic Staples

If your local grocery store doesn't carry certain ethnic spices or ingredients, you may be able to find them on the Internet or at specialty shops. Just make sure to stock up on shelf-stable necessities so you can make these dishes whenever you like.

1. Remove the skin and bones from chicken breasts.

2. Heat ½ cup of the coconut milk and the green curry paste in a medium skillet over medium heat; stir until well blended. Add the chicken and sauté for 10 minutes.

3. Place the chicken breasts into the slow cooker. Stir in the remaining coconut milk, bamboo shoots, fish sauce, and erythritol.

4. Cover and cook on a low setting for 6–7 hours.

5. Stir in the mint and chili peppers. Cover and cook an additional 30 minutes.

Cauliflower and Ham Chowder

Serve with an array of pickled vegetables to offset the creamy sweet flavor of this soup.

INGREDIENTS | SERVES 6

1 cup canned full-fat coconut milk
1 tablespoon tapioca flour
2 cups diced ham
3 cups chopped fresh cauliflower
1 small white onion, finely chopped
1 cup grated Swiss cheese
2 cups water
1 cup heavy cream

1. Mix the coconut milk and tapioca flour in the slow cooker.

2. Add the ham, cauliflower, onion, Swiss cheese, and water to the slow cooker.

3. Cover and cook on a low setting for 8–9 hours.

4. Ten minutes before serving, stir in the cream.

The Squash Bowl

Use squash as a soup bowl! Many small squashes make excellent complements to soups and stews. Cut them in half, remove the seeds, and prebake in the microwave or oven. Ladle your soup or stew into the squash for a festive look.

Hamburger Vegetable Soup

It's easy to adapt this soup to suit your taste buds. Try adding some fresh herbs such as parsley, or use ground pork or turkey instead of beef. A topping of freshly grated Parmesan adds flavor and makes a great presentation, too.

INGREDIENTS | SERVES 6

½ pound ground beef

6 cups sugar-free beef broth

3 medium fresh tomatoes, diced

1 large yellow onion, chopped

½ cup chopped celery

½ teaspoon salt

½ teaspoon black pepper

1 cup chopped fresh asparagus

1 cup fresh green beans

1. Brown the ground beef in a medium skillet over medium-high heat, breaking and crumbling into smaller pieces, about 7–10 minutes. Drain off grease.

2. Place the ground beef, beef broth, tomatoes, onion, celery, salt, and pepper in slow cooker. Cover and cook on a low setting for 6 hours.

3. Add the asparagus and green beans. Cover and cook on low 1–2 more hours before serving. If desired, serve with freshly grated Parmesan cheese, or a scoop of sour cream.

Thicken It Up

To create a thicker soup, remove some of the cooked vegetables from the broth and purée them in a blender, then stir them back into the soup. Or add full-fat coconut milk for an even richer soup.

French Countryside Chicken and Pork Stew

Top with chopped parsley and a dollop of sour cream right before serving.

INGREDIENTS | SERVES 4

3 pounds pork chops

4 chicken breasts

2 tablespoons olive oil

10 pearl onions, peeled

4 cloves garlic, minced

2 cups sugar-free beef broth

¼ cup sugar-free chicken stock

2 tablespoons Dijon mustard

4 ounces (½ cup) fresh mushrooms, quartered

1 teaspoon warm water

1 teaspoon tapioca flour

Preparing Pearl Onions

When using pearl onions, cook them first in boiling water for 3 minutes. Plunge them into cold water. Remove them from the water and cut off the ends before easily removing the skin.

1. Remove the bones from the pork and cut the meat into ½" cubes. Remove the bones and skin from the chicken and discard; cut the chicken into ½" cubes.

2. Heat olive oil in a large skillet over medium-high heat. Sauté the pork, chicken, onions, and garlic until the meat is browned, about 7 minutes.

3. Drain off grease and add mixture to the slow cooker.

4. Combine beef broth, chicken stock, and mustard in a medium bowl and pour mixture into the slow cooker. Add mushrooms on top.

5. Cover and cook on a low setting for 8–9 hours.

6. About 30 minutes before serving, make a paste of the warm water and tapioca flour; add to the slow cooker, stirring well. Cook uncovered, stirring occasionally, until a gravy develops.

7. Serve with desired garnishes.

Chili Coconut Chicken

The coconut milk provides a nice balance to the red chilies. Serve this over Fried Cauliflower "Rice" or Mashed Cauliflower (see recipes in Chapter 11).

INGREDIENTS | SERVES 4

½ teaspoon black mustard seeds

½ teaspoon cumin seeds

½ teaspoon coriander seeds

3 tablespoons coconut oil

8 curry leaves

1 medium red onion, finely chopped

2 teaspoons Ginger-Garlic Paste (see sidebar recipe)

3 dried red chilies, roughly pounded

½ teaspoon turmeric powder

Salt, to taste

1½ pounds boneless, skinless chicken, cubed

Water, as needed

1 cup full-fat canned coconut milk

Ginger-Garlic Paste

Remove the stems from 2 serrano green chilies. (The chilies are optional; omit if you like a milder paste.) Place chilies, ½ cup peeled fresh gingerroot, ½ cup peeled garlic cloves, and 1 tablespoon cold water in a food processor and purée to form a smooth paste. Add no more than 1 tablespoon of water to help form a smooth consistency. Store the paste in an airtight jar in the refrigerator. The paste will keep for up to 2 weeks in the refrigerator.

1. In a small skillet over medium heat, dry-roast the mustard seeds, cumin seeds, and coriander seeds. When the spices release their aroma, about 3 minutes, remove from heat and let cool. In a spice grinder, grind to a coarse powder. Set aside.

2. In a large skillet, heat the coconut oil over medium heat. Add the curry leaves and the onions; sauté for about 1 minute.

3. Add the Ginger-Garlic Paste and dried red chilies. Sauté over medium heat until the onions are well browned and the oil begins to separate from the sides of the onion mixture, about 8 minutes. (You can also use ½ cup jarred curry paste, but the results would be slightly different because of the strong flavor of the garam masala in most curry pastes.)

4. Add the ground mustard, cumin, and coriander seeds, turmeric powder, and salt; sauté for 1 minute.

5. Add the chicken pieces; mix well and transfer into a 3–4-quart slow cooker. You can add up to ¼ cup of water if the ground spices don't incorporate as well as you'd like, although not necessary.

6. Cover and cook on high for 2–3 hours, or on low for 4–6 hours, or until the chicken is cooked through.

7. During the last 30 minutes, add the coconut milk and simmer. Serve hot.

Mixed Vegetables in Coconut Sauce

*Use your choice of seasonal vegetables to make this dish. Serve with Turnip Fries or Mashed Cauliflower
(see recipes in Chapter 11), or over roasted spaghetti squash and your choice of any hot pickle.*

INGREDIENTS | SERVES 4

1 cup unsweetened desiccated coconut

1 tablespoon toasted cumin seeds

2 green serrano chilies, seeded

Water, as needed

2 small carrots, peeled and chopped

½ pound frozen cut green beans, thawed

¼ cup Coconut Yogurt (see Chapter 12)

¼ cup sour cream

½ teaspoon turmeric powder

Salt, to taste

1 tablespoon coconut oil

1 teaspoon black mustard seeds

8 curry leaves

1. In a food processor, grind the coconut, cumin seeds, and green chilies along with a few tablespoons of water to make a thick paste. Set aside.

2. In a slow cooker, combine the carrots, green beans, and 1½ cups of water. Cover and cook on high for 1½ hours, or on low for 3 hours, or until the vegetables are soft. Drain off any remaining water.

3. Add the yogurt, sour cream, reserved coconut paste, turmeric, and salt to the vegetables. Simmer until the vegetables are completely cooked through, another 45 minutes on high or 1½ hours or low. When cooked through, turn off the heat and set aside.

4. In a small skillet, heat the coconut oil over medium heat. Add the mustard seeds and curry leaves. When the seeds begin to crackle, remove from heat and pour over the cooked vegetables. Serve hot.

Lamb Vindaloo

You can also prepare this with pork or beef; adjust seasonings to taste.
(The cooking times will stay the same.)

INGREDIENTS | SERVES 4

¾ cup rice vinegar

¼ cup water

1 teaspoon black peppercorns, roughly pounded

1 tablespoon minced garlic

2 teaspoons red chili powder

2 green serrano chilies, minced

1½ pounds boneless lean lamb, cubed

3 tablespoons light olive oil

1 tablespoon grated gingerroot

1 large red onion, peeled and finely chopped

6 whole dried red chilies, roughly pounded

1 (1") cinnamon stick

½ teaspoon turmeric powder

Salt, to taste

Selecting Lamb

Color can be a great help when buying lamb. Younger lamb is pinkish red with a velvety texture. It should have a thin layer of white fat surrounding it. If the meat is much darker in color, it means that the lamb is older and flavored more strongly.

1. In the slow cooker insert, combine the rice vinegar, water, black peppercorns, garlic, red chili powder, and green chilies. Add the lamb and coat evenly with the marinade. Refrigerate, covered, for 1 hour.

2. In a deep pan, heat the oil over medium heat. Add the gingerroot and sauté for about 10 seconds. Add the onion and sauté for about 7–8 minutes or until golden brown.

3. Add the dried red chilies, cinnamon stick, and turmeric powder; sauté for 20 seconds.

4. Remove the lamb pieces from the marinade. Add the lamb to the pan with onions and sauté on high heat for about 10 minutes or until the lamb is browned and the oil starts to separate from the mixture.

5. Transfer the browned lamb back to the slow cooker. Mix with the marinade and salt. Cover and cook on high for 4–5 hours, or on low for 8–10 hours, or until the lamb is cooked through and tender. Serve hot.

Spicy Shrimp and Cheese Dip

Cooking tip: If the dip is too thick, add coconut milk or heavy cream in half-cup increments until it's the consistency you like. This dip is heavenly with the addition of 1 cup chopped cooked scallops.

INGREDIENTS | SERVES 12–24 AS AN APPETIZER

2 slices sugar-free bacon

1 cup popcorn shrimp (not the breaded kind), cooked

2 medium yellow onions, diced

2 cloves garlic, minced

1 medium tomato, diced

3 cups shredded Monterey jack cheese

¼ teaspoon sugar-free hot sauce

¼ teaspoon cayenne pepper

¼ teaspoon black pepper

Cleaning

Use a rough sponge to remove any dried-on food from the slow cooker when cleaning it. A scouring pad could scratch the surface, creating a place for bacteria to grow.

1. Cook the bacon in a medium skillet over medium heat until crisp, about 5–10 minutes. Keep grease in pan. Lay the bacon on a paper towel to cool.

2. When cool, crumble the bacon with your fingers.

3. If the shrimp is not precooked, boil it in water for 10 minutes. Drain and cool.

4. Add the onion and garlic to the bacon drippings in the skillet and sauté over medium-low heat until they are soft and fragrant, about 10 minutes.

5. Combine all the ingredients in the slow cooker; stir well. Cook covered on a low setting for 1–2 hours, or until the cheese is fully melted.

Creamy Pecan Beef Dip

Try this unique dip at your next gathering. Serve with bell pepper wedges and cucumber rounds. Provide plenty of veggies—this dip goes quickly!

INGREDIENTS | SERVES 6

3 ounces sliced smoked beef
2 tablespoons finely chopped onion
½ cup finely chopped pecans
2 tablespoons minced green pepper
8 ounces cream cheese
½ cup sour cream
2 tablespoons heavy cream
⅛ teaspoon white pepper

1. Finely shred the smoked beef.

2. Combine all ingredients in the slow cooker.

3. Cover and heat on a low setting for 2–3 hours or until dip bubbles at edges. Do not overheat.

Artichoke Dip

For a truly unique appetizer, dollop this dip on top of Parmesan Chips (see Chapter 13). Alternatively, use bell pepper strips and celery sticks to scoop and add crunch.

INGREDIENTS | SERVES 6 AS AN APPETIZER

⅓ cup mayonnaise

½ cup grated Parmesan cheese

⅓ cup full-fat sour cream

1 clove garlic, finely minced

6 ounces (1½ cups) marinated artichoke hearts, chopped into penny-sized pieces

1. Combine the mayonnaise, Parmesan, sour cream, and garlic. Mix in the chopped artichoke hearts.

2. Place the mixture in the slow cooker, cover, and cook on a low setting for 1 hour. Mix periodically while it is cooking to ensure that all ingredients combine and meld together.

Storage Tip

Store the slow cooker with the lid alongside instead of on top to prevent the chance that mold will grow if you don't use it for several weeks.

Appendix A: Shopping List

FATS AND OILS

- Butter
- Coconut oil
- Coconut butter
- Olive oil
- Olives
- Avocados
- Avocado oil
- Coconut flakes (unsweetened)
- Full-fat coconut milk

PROTEIN

- Poultry: chicken, turkey, duck (free-range is best)
- Meat: beef, veal, venison, bison, lamb (grass-fed is best)
- Pork: Pork loin, ham, pork chops (humanely treated, pastured is best; make sure ham contains no sugar)
- Eggs
- Bacon
- Sausage
- Deli meat: prosciutto, pepperoni, turkey, roast beef, ham (make sure there is no added sugar)
- Fresh fish: cod, salmon, halibut, mackerel, herring, sardines, tuna, anchovies (wild-caught is best)
- Shellfish: shrimp, crab, lobster, scallops, mussels, oysters, clams
- Canned tuna
- Canned salmon

DAIRY PRODUCTS

- Heavy cream
- Sour cream
- Ricotta cheese
- Cottage cheese
- Cream cheese
- Cheddar cheese
- Parmesan cheese
- Pepper jack cheese
- Mozzarella cheese
- Asiago cheese

FRUITS

- Blackberries
- Blueberries
- Raspberries
- Granny Smith apples
- Lemons

VEGETABLES

- Bell peppers
- Cucumbers
- Broccoli
- Eggplant
- Spinach
- Baby kale
- Cabbage
- Cauliflower
- Lettuce (iceberg and romaine)
- Onions
- Garlic
- Scallions
- Shallots
- Mushrooms
- Celery
- Brussels sprouts
- Asparagus
- Zucchini
- Spaghetti squash
- Canned whole tomatoes
- Fire-roasted diced tomatoes

NUTS, NUT BUTTERS, AND SEEDS

- Almonds
- Almond butter
- Cashews
- Cashew butter
- Pecans
- Pistachio nuts
- Macadamia nuts
- Chia seeds
- Peanuts
- Peanut butter
- Walnuts
- Pumpkin seeds
- Sunflower seeds

CONDIMENTS

- Pickles
- Mustard
- White vinegar
- Apple cider vinegar
- Hot sauce

SWEETENERS AND EXTRACTS

- Erythritol (granulated and powdered)
- Stevia (liquid and granulated)
- Vanilla extract
- Almond extract
- Orange extract
- Peppermint extract

MISCELLANEOUS

- Pork rinds
- Dark chocolate
- Unsweetened cocoa powder
- Whey protein powder (sugar-free—low net carbohydrates)

Appendix B: Sample Meal Plans

Week 1:

Sunday
Breakfast: Pumpkin Pie Smoothie (Chapter 16)
Lunch: BLT Salad (Chapter 10)
Dinner: "Spaghetti" and Spicy Meatballs with Garlicky Green Beans (Chapters 8 and 11)
Dessert: Chocolate Brownies (Chapter 14)
Snack: Pizza Bites (Chapter 13)

Monday
Breakfast: Sausage Quiche (Chapter 6)
Lunch: Taco Salad (Chapter 10)
Dinner: Stuffed Chicken Breast (Chapter 8)
Dessert: Lemon Mug Cake with Lemon Icing (Chapter 14)
Snack: Peanut Butter Fat Bombs (Chapter 15)

Tuesday
Breakfast: Western Scrambled Eggs (Chapter 6)
Lunch: Leftover Sausage Quiche (Chapter 6)
Dinner: Creamy Chicken Zoodles (Chapter 8)
Dessert: Pistachio Pudding (Chapter 14)
Snack: Lemon Cheesecake Fat Bombs (Chapter 15)

Wednesday
Breakfast: Coconut Chia Smoothie (Chapter 16)
Lunch: Cobb Salad (Chapter 10)
Dinner: Pepperoni Meat-za with Turnip Fries (Chapters 8 and 11)
Dessert: Chocolate Mug Cake (Chapter 14)
Snack: Pumpkin Pie Coconut Crisps (Chapter 13)

Thursday
Breakfast: Spicy Sausage Egg Cups (Chapter 6)
Lunch: "Mac" 'n' Cheese (Chapter 7)
Dinner: Bacon-Wrapped Chicken with Avocado and Cilantro Salad (Chapters 8 and 11)
Dessert: Snickerdoodle Cookies (Chapter 14)
Snack: Stuffed Olives (Chapter 13)

Friday
Breakfast: Leftover Spicy Sausage Egg Cups (Chapter 6)
Lunch: Meatball "Sub" (Chapter 7)
Dinner: Shepherd's Pie (Chapter 8)
Dessert: Chocolate Ice Cream (Chapter 14)
Snack: Cocoa Coconut Butter Fat Bombs (Chapter 15)

Saturday
Breakfast: Bacon-and-Egg-Stuffed Avocados (Chapter 6)
Lunch: Pepperoni Pizza Casserole (Chapter 7)
Dinner: Spinach and Prosciutto Salad (Chapter 10)
Dessert: Walnut Blondies (Chapter 14)
Snack: Parmesan Chips (Chapter 13)

Week 2:

Sunday
Breakfast: Ham, Cheese, and Egg Casserole (Chapter 6)
Lunch: Spinach, Feta, and Apple Salad (Chapter 10)
Dinner: Stuffed Pork Tenderloin (Chapter 8)
Dessert: Chocolate Brownie Cheesecake (Chapter 14)
Snack: Kale and Brazil Nut Smoothie (Chapter 16)

Monday
Breakfast: Bacon-Wrapped Egg Cups (Chapter 6)
Lunch: Pumpkin Cream Soup (Chapter 9)
Dinner: Shrimp Scampi (Chapter 8) over baked spaghetti squash
Dessert: Leftover Chocolate Brownie Cheesecake (Chapter 14)
Snack: Almond Butter Fat Bombs (Chapter 15)

Tuesday
Breakfast: Leftover Ham, Cheese, and Egg Casserole (Chapter 6)
Lunch: Bacon-Wrapped Chicken Bites and Cole Slaw (Chapters 13 and 11)
Dinner: Leftover Pumpkin Cream Soup and Salmon and Avocado Salad (Chapters 9 and 10)
Dessert: Spiced Chocolate Smoothie (Chapter 16)
Snack: Pepperoni Chips (Chapter 13)

Wednesday
Breakfast: Leftover Bacon-Wrapped Egg Cups (Chapter 6)
Lunch: Leftover Stuffed Pork Tenderloin (Chapter 8)
Dinner: "Spaghetti" and Spicy Meatballs with Marinara Sauce (Chapters 8 and 9)
Dessert: Walnut Blondies with Coconut Whipped Cream (Chapter 14)
Snack: Leftover Almond Butter Fat Bombs (Chapter 15)

Thursday
Breakfast: Peanut Butter Pancakes (Chapter 12)
Lunch: Stuffed Avocados (Chapter 7)
Dinner: Gorgonzola Steak Salad (Chapter 10)
Dessert: Orange Coconut Smoothie (Chapter 16)
Snack: Guacamole (Chapter 13) with celery sticks

Friday
Breakfast: Almond Butter Muffins (Chapter 6)
Lunch: Breadless BLT (Chapter 7)
Dinner: Ground Pork Stir-Fry (Chapter 8)
Dessert: Chocolate Fudge Sauce (Chapter 14) over Chocolate Ice Cream (Chapter 14)
Snack: Lemon Cheesecake Fat Bombs (Chapter 15)

Saturday
Breakfast: Eggs Benedict (Chapter 6) with Hollandaise Sauce (Chapter 9)
Lunch: Leftover Ground Pork Stir-Fry (Chapter 8)
Dinner: Stuffed Green Peppers (Chapter 8)
Dessert: Chocolate Chip Cookies (Chapter 14)
Snack: Leftover Almond Butter Muffins (Chapter 6)

Week 3:

Sunday
Breakfast: Scrambled Eggs with Bacon (Chapter 6)
Lunch: Fried Chicken (Chapter 7)
Dinner: Meaty Chili (Chapter 17)
Dessert: Peanut Butter Cookies with Coconut Whipped Cream (Chapter 14)
Snack: Jalapeño Poppers with Ranch Dressing (Chapters 13 and 9)

Monday
Breakfast: Coconut Yogurt (Chapter 12) with ¼ cup strawberries and 2 tablespoons almonds
Lunch: Chilled Spicy Avocado Soup (Chapter 9)
Dinner: Leftover Fried Chicken (Chapter 7) with Mashed Cauliflower (Chapter 11)
Dessert: Banana Nut Smoothie (Chapter 16)
Snack: Green Deviled Eggs (Chapter 13)

Tuesday
Breakfast: Triple Green Smoothie (Chapter 16)
Lunch: Leftover Meaty Chili (Chapter 17)
Dinner: Tomato Cream Soup (Chapter 12) and Cheesy Broccoli (Chapter 11)
Dessert: Blueberry Fat Bomb (Chapter 15)
Snack: Leftover Peanut Butter Cookies (Chapter 14)

Wednesday
Breakfast: Fried egg and Bacon Hash (Chapter 6)
Lunch: Cheeseburger Salad (Chapter 10)
Dinner: Stuffed Portobello Mushrooms (Chapter 12)
Dessert: Chocolate Mug Cake (Chapter 14)
Snack: Parmesan Chips (Chapter 13)

Thursday
Breakfast: Cinnamon Noatmeal (Chapter 12)
Lunch: Taco Bowls (Chapter 8)
Dinner: Stuffed Chicken Breast (Chapter 8) and Zoodles with Avocado Pesto (Chapter 12)
Dessert: Prosciutto Chips (Chapter 13)
Snack: Vanilla Macadamia Fat Bombs (Chapter 15)

Friday
Breakfast: Chocolate Almond Smoothie (Chapter 16)
Lunch: Deli Roll-Ups (Chapter 7)
Dinner: Bunless Bacon Burgers (Chapter 8) and Cole Slaw (Chapter 11)
Dessert: Pecan-Crusted Cheesecake (Chapter 14)
Snack: Tuna Salad and Cucumber Bites (Chapter 13)

Saturday
Breakfast: Pumpkin Donut Holes (Chapter 14)
Lunch: Chef Salad (Chapter 10)
Dinner: Zucchini Chicken Alfredo (Chapter 8)
Dessert: Leftover Pecan-Crusted Cheesecake (Chapter 14)
Snack: Deviled Eggs (Chapter 13)

Week 4:

Sunday
Breakfast: Ham, Cheese, and Egg Casserole (Chapter 6)
Lunch: Spinach and Tuna Salad (Chapter 10)
Dinner: Meatloaf (Chapter 8) and Buttery Garlic Spinach (Chapter 11)
Dessert: Mint Chocolate Chip Ice Cream (Chapter 14)
Snack: Maple Fat Bombs (Chapter 15)

Monday
Breakfast: Scrambled Eggs with Bacon (Chapter 6)
Lunch: Chicken Soup (Chapter 9)
Dinner: Leftover Meatloaf (Chapter 8) and Buttery Garlic Spinach (Chapter 11)
Dessert: Leftover Mint Chocolate Chip Ice Cream (Chapter 14)
Snack: Pepperoni Cheese Bites (Chapter 13)

Tuesday
Breakfast: Leftover Ham, Cheese, and Egg Casserole (Chapter 6)
Lunch: Bacon Cheddar Soup (Chapter 9)
Dinner: Kale and Salmon Salad (Chapter 10)
Dessert: Leftover Maple Fat Bombs (Chapter 15)
Snack: Coffee Coconut Berry Smoothie (Chapter 12)

Wednesday
Breakfast: Green Smoothie (Chapter 16)
Lunch: Bacon and Broccoli Salad (Chapter 10)
Dinner: Baked Salmon with Garlic Aioli (Chapter 8)

Dessert: Chocolate Mousse (Chapter 13)
Snack: ¼ cup blackberries and Coconut Yogurt (Chapter 12)

Thursday
Breakfast: Almond Butter Muffins (Chapter 6)
Lunch: Avocado and Walnut Salad (Chapter 12)
Dinner: Taco Bowls (Chapter 8)
Dessert: Cinnamon Bun Fat Bombs (Chapter 15)
Snack: Parmesan Chips (Chapter 13)

Friday
Breakfast: Cinnamon Noatmeal (Chapter 12)
Lunch: Roast Beef Lettuce Wraps (Chapter 7)
Dinner: Spicy Chicken and Avocado Casserole (Chapter 7)
Dessert: Walnut Blondies (Chapter 14)
Snack: Leftover Almond Butter Muffins (Chapter 6)

Saturday
Breakfast: Eggs Benedict (Chapter 6)
Lunch: Leftover Spicy Chicken and Avocado Casserole (Chapter 7)
Dinner: Chicken Cordon Bleu Casserole (Chapter 7)
Dessert: Leftover Walnut Blondies (Chapter 14)
Snack: Mixed Nut Butter Bombs (Chapter 15)

Week 5:

Sunday
Breakfast: Spinach and Mozzarella Egg Bake (Chapter 6)
Lunch: Tuna and Egg Salad (Chapter 7)
Dinner: Stuffed Green Peppers (Chapter 8)
Dessert: Coconut Peppermint Fat Bombs (Chapter 15)
Snack: Pizza Bites (Chapter 13)

Monday
Breakfast: Scrambled eggs and Bacon Hash (Chapter 6)
Lunch: Creamy Broccoli Soup (Chapter 9)
Dinner: Stuffed Pork Tenderloin (Chapter 8) and Roasted Broccoli with Parmesan (Chapter 11)
Dessert: Leftover Coconut Peppermint Fat Bombs (Chapter 15)
Snack: Monkey Salad (Chapter 10)

Tuesday
Breakfast: Leftover Spinach and Mozzarella Egg Bake (Chapter 6)
Lunch: Portobello Pizzas (Chapter 7)
Dinner: Leftover Stuffed Green Peppers (Chapter 8)
Dessert: Lime and Coconut Smoothie (Chapter 16)
Snack: Guacamole (Chapter 13) and cucumber slices

Wednesday
Breakfast: Carrot Asparagus Green Smoothie (Chapter 16)
Lunch: Turkey Avocado Rolls (Chapter 7)

Dinner: Bacon Spinach Salad with Creamy Ranch Dressing (Chapter 10)
Dessert: Snickerdoodle Cookies (Chapter 14)
Snack: Turnip Fries (Chapter 11)

Thursday
Breakfast: Western Scrambled Eggs (Chapter 6)
Lunch: Avocado Egg Salad (Chapter 10)
Dinner: Baked Zucchini (Chapter 12)
Dessert: Lemon Mug Cake with Lemon Icing (Chapter 14)
Snack: Calming Cucumber Smoothie (Chapter 16)

Friday
Breakfast: Veggie Omelet (Chapter 12)
Lunch: Meatball "Sub" (Chapter 7)
Dinner: Grilled chicken breast and Cheesy Bacon Brussels Sprouts (Chapter 11)
Dessert: Leftover Snickerdoodle Cookies (Chapter 14)
Snack: Pumpkin Fat Bombs (Chapter 15)

Saturday
Breakfast: Peanut Butter Pancakes (Chapter 12)
Lunch: Gorgonzola Steak Salad (Chapter 10)
Dinner: Ground Pork Stir-Fry (Chapter 8)
Dessert: Chocolate Chia Pudding (Chapter 12)
Snack: Cashew Butter Cup Fat Bombs (Chapter 15)

Week 6:

Sunday
Breakfast: Spicy Sausage Egg Cups (Chapter 6)
Lunch: Spinach, Feta, and Apple Salad (Chapter 10)
Dinner: Meaty Chili (Chapter 17)
Dessert: Snickerdoodle Cookies (Chapter 14)
Snack: Ginger Strawberry Smoothie (Chapter 16)

Monday
Breakfast: Coconut Yogurt (Chapter 12) with ½ cup almonds and ¼ cup blackberries
Lunch: Deli Roll-Ups (Chapter 7)
Dinner: Taco Salad (Chapter 10)
Dessert: Leftover Snickerdoodle Cookies (Chapter 14)
Snack: Leftover Spicy Sausage Egg Cups (Chapter 6)

Tuesday
Breakfast: Banana Nut Smoothie (Chapter 16)
Lunch: Leftover Meaty Chili (Chapter 17)
Dinner: Shrimp Scampi (Chapter 8)
Dessert: Lemon Cheesecake Fat Bombs (Chapter 15)
Snack: Stuffed Olives (Chapter 13)

Wednesday
Breakfast: Scrambled Eggs with Bacon (Chapter 6)
Lunch: Leftover Shrimp Scampi (Chapter 8)
Dinner: Creamy Spaghetti Squash (Chapter 12) and grilled salmon
Dessert: Orange Coconut Smoothie (Chapter 16)

Snack: Leftover Lemon Cheesecake Fat Bombs (Chapter 15)

Thursday
Breakfast: Crustless Quiche (Chapter 12)
Lunch: Portobello Pizzas (Chapter 7)
Dinner: Chicken Cordon Bleu Casserole (Chapter 7)
Dessert: Chocolate Brownie Cheesecake (Chapter 14)
Snack: Pepperoni Chips (Chapter 13)

Friday
Breakfast: Coconut Chia Smoothie (Chapter 16)
Lunch: Leftover Crustless Quiche (Chapter 12) and ¼ cup sliced cherry tomatoes
Dinner: Bacon-Wrapped Chicken (Chapter 8) and Fried Cauliflower "Rice" (Chapter 11)
Dessert: Chocolate Chip Cookies (Chapter 14)
Snack: Tuna Salad and Cucumber Bites (Chapter 13)

Saturday
Breakfast: Honeydew and Avocado Smoothie (Chapter 16)
Lunch: Leftover Chicken Cordon Bleu Casserole (Chapter 7)
Dinner: Bunless Bacon Burgers (Chapter 8) and Parmesan Chips (Chapter 13)
Dessert: Leftover Chocolate Brownie Cheesecake (Chapter 14)
Snack: Avocado Fat Bomb Smoothie (Chapter 15)

Week 7:

Sunday
Breakfast: Bacon-and-Egg-Stuffed Avocados (Chapter 6)
Lunch: Chicken Soup (Chapter 9)
Dinner: Cauliflower Casserole (Chapter 12)
Dessert: Pistachio Pudding (Chapter 14)
Snack: 2 tablespoons cashew butter mixed with 2 tablespoons unsweetened coconut flakes on celery sticks

Monday
Breakfast: Coconut Yogurt (Chapter 12) with ½ cup sliced almonds
Lunch: Leftover Cauliflower Casserole (Chapter 12) and Chicken Soup (Chapter 9)
Dinner: Cobb Salad (Chapter 10)
Dessert: Chocolate Ice Cream (Chapter 14)
Snack: ½ cup grape tomatoes and Blue Cheese Dressing (Chapter 9)

Tuesday
Breakfast: Pumpkin Pie Smoothie (Chapter 16)
Lunch: Bacon Cheddar Soup (Chapter 9)
Dinner: Zoodles with Avocado Pesto (Chapter 12)
Dessert: Leftover Pistachio Pudding (Chapter 14)
Snack: Green Deviled Eggs (Chapter 13)

Wednesday
Breakfast: Cinnamon Noatmeal (Chapter 12)
Lunch: Leftover Zoodles with Avocado Pesto (Chapter 12) and Parmesan Chips (Chapter 13)
Dinner: Pumpkin Cream Soup (Chapter 9) with sour cream and cilantro
Dessert: Leftover Chocolate Ice Cream (Chapter 14)
Snack: Monkey Salad (Chapter 10)

Thursday
Breakfast: Coconut Cream Dream Smoothie (Chapter 16)
Lunch: Cheeseburger Salad (Chapter 10)
Dinner: Ricotta-Stuffed Eggplant (Chapter 12)
Dessert: Coconut Whipped Cream (Chapter 14) with ½ cup strawberries
Snack: ¼ cup walnuts

Friday
Breakfast: Ham, Cheese, and Egg Casserole (Chapter 6)
Lunch: BLT Salad (Chapter 10)
Dinner: Turkey burger and Turnip Fries (Chapter 11) with Garlic Aioli (Chapter 9)
Dessert: Coconut Peppermint Fat Bombs (Chapter 15)
Snack: Calming Cucumber Smoothie (Chapter 16)

Saturday
Breakfast: Avocado Fat Bomb Smoothie (Chapter 15)
Lunch: Leftover Ham, Cheese, and Egg Casserole (Chapter 6)
Dinner: Pepperoni Meat-Za (Chapter 8)
Dessert: Pumpkin Donut Holes (Chapter 14)
Snack: 1 cup Coconut Yogurt (Chapter 12) mixed with cinnamon

Week 8:

Sunday
Breakfast: Scrambled eggs and Bacon Hash (Chapter 6)
Lunch: Creamy Broccoli Soup (Chapter 9)
Dinner: Spicy Chicken and Avocado Casserole (Chapter 7)
Dessert: Chocolate Mousse (Chapter 13)
Snack: Jalapeño Poppers (Chapter 13)

Monday
Breakfast: Coconut Chia Smoothie (Chapter 16)
Lunch: Leftover Bacon Hash (Chapter 6) and Cheesy Broccoli (Chapter 11)
Dinner: Avocado and Cilantro Salad (Chapter 11)
Dessert: Vanilla Macadamia Fat Bomb (Chapter 15)
Snack: 1 cup celery sticks and Avocado Italian Dressing (Chapter 9)

Tuesday
Breakfast: Crustless Quiche (Chapter 12)
Lunch: Leftover Spicy Chicken and Avocado Casserole (Chapter 7)
Dinner: Stuffed Portobello Mushrooms (Chapter 12)
Dessert: Leftover Chocolate Mousse (Chapter 13)
Snack: ½ cup blueberries with ½ cup pecans

Wednesday
Breakfast: Kale and Brazil Nut Smoothie (Chapter 16)
Lunch: Leftover Crustless Quiche (Chapter 12)
Dinner: "Mac" 'n' Cheese (Chapter 7)
Dessert: Raspberry Cheesecake Fat Bombs (Chapter 15)
Snack: ½ cup sliced bell peppers and Blue Cheese Dressing (Chapter 9)

Thursday
Breakfast: Almond Butter Muffins (Chapter 6)
Lunch: Meatball "Sub" (Chapter 7)
Dinner: Chicken Cordon Bleu Casserole (Chapter 7)
Dessert: Chocolate Mug Cake (Chapter 14)
Snack: Leftover Raspberry Cheesecake Fat Bombs (Chapter 15)

Friday
Breakfast: Peanut Butter Pancakes (Chapter 12)
Lunch: Leftover "Mac" 'n' Cheese (Chapter 7) and Cole Slaw (Chapter 11)
Dinner: Kale and Salmon Salad (Chapter 10)
Dessert: Lemon Mug Cake with Lemon Icing (Chapter 14)
Snack: Leftover Almond Butter Muffins (Chapter 6)

Saturday
Breakfast: Eggs Benedict (Chapter 6) and Hollandaise Sauce (Chapter 9)
Lunch: Leftover Chicken Cordon Bleu Casserole (Chapter 7)
Dinner: Meatloaf (Chapter 8) and Mashed Cauliflower (Chapter 11)
Dessert: Ginger Strawberry Smoothie (Chapter 16)
Snack: Mixed Nut Butter Bombs (Chapter 15)

Vegetarian Meal Plan:

Sunday

Breakfast: Peanut Butter Pancakes (Chapter 12)
Lunch: Avocado Egg Salad (Chapter 10)
Dinner: Cauliflower Casserole (Chapter 12)
Dessert: Chocolate Brownies (Chapter 14)
Snack: Carrot Asparagus Green Smoothie
(Chapter 16)

Monday

Breakfast: ¼ cup raspberries and Coconut Yogurt
(Chapter 12)
Lunch: Leftover Cauliflower Casserole (Chapter
12)
Dinner: Crustless Quiche (Chapter 12)
Dessert: Leftover Chocolate Brownies (Chapter
14)
Snack: ½ cup almonds

Tuesday

Breakfast: Veggie Omelet (Chapter 12)
Lunch: Chilled Spicy Avocado Soup (Chapter 9)
(swap chicken broth with vegetable broth)
Dinner: Ricotta-Stuffed Eggplant (Chapter 12)
Dessert: Spiced Chocolate Smoothie (Chapter 16)
Snack: Monkey Salad (Chapter 10)

Wednesday

Breakfast: Cinnamon Noatmeal (Chapter 12)
Lunch: Leftover Crustless Quiche (Chapter 12)
Dinner: Stuffed Portobello Mushrooms (Chapter
12)
Dessert: Pumpkin Pie Coconut Crisps (Chapter 13)
Snack: Coffee Coconut Berry Smoothie (Chapter
12)

Thursday

Breakfast: 2 fried eggs and ½ sliced avocado
Lunch: Leftover Ricotta-Stuffed Eggplant (Chapter
12)
Dinner: Leftover Chilled Spicy Avocado Soup
(Chapter 9) and Mexican Cauliflower "Rice"
(Chapter 11)
Dessert: Cocoa Coconut Butter Fat Bombs
(Chapter 15)
Snack: Almond Berry Smoothie (Chapter 16)

Friday

Breakfast: Green Smoothie (Chapter 16)
Lunch: Tomato Cream Soup (Chapter 12)
Dinner: Avocado and Walnut Salad (Chapter 12)
Dessert: Chocolate Chia Pudding (Chapter 12)
Snack: Raspberry Cheesecake Fat Bombs
(Chapter 15)

Saturday

Breakfast: Almond Butter Muffins (Chapter 6)
Lunch: Creamy Broccoli Soup (Chapter 9) (swap
chicken broth with vegetable broth)
Dinner: Baked Zucchini (Chapter 12)
Dessert: Maple Fat Bombs (Chapter 15)
Snack: Roasted Broccoli with Parmesan (Chapter
11)

Appendix C: Resources

Boston Children's Hospital

300 Longwood Avenue
Boston, MA 02115
(617) 355-6815
www.childrenshospital.org
Boston Children's Hospital has a Pediatric
Epilepsy Program that provides support for
children with epilepsy. Their program is rated
as a Level 4 Epilepsy Center by the National
Association of Epilepsy Centers because they
deliver an extremely high level of care that
includes the use of the ketogenic diet.

Children's Hospital Los Angeles

4650 Sunset Blvd.
Los Angeles, CA 90027
(323) 660-2450
www.chla.org
Children's Hospital Los Angeles specializes in
pediatrics and uses the classic ketogenic diet
and modified ketogenic diet as part of their
epilepsy treatment program.

Keto Calculator

http://keto-calculator.ankerl.com/
Easily calculate your macronutrient ratios for the
ketogenic diet with this online diet calculator.

The Charlie Foundation

515 Ocean Avenue
#602N
Santa Monica, CA 90402
(310) 393-2347
www.charliefoundation.org
The Charlie Foundation for Ketogenic Therapies
provides information and dietary therapies
for people with epilepsy, other neurological
disorders, and cancer.

The Institute for Functional Medicine

505 S. 336th Street
Suite 500
Federal Way, WA 98003
(800) 228-0622
www.functionalmedicine.org
The goal of the Institute for Functional Medicine
is to reverse chronic disease and advance
knowledge by providing information and
education about functional medicine.

The UltraWellness Center

Dr. Mark Hyman
55 Pittsfield Road
Suite 9
Lenox Commons, Lenox, MA 01240
(413) 637-9991
www.ultrawellnesscenter.com
Dr. Mark Hyman is one of the leaders
in functional medicine. He founded the
UltraWellness Center in Lenox, Massachusetts,
and has authored several books.

Standard U.S./Metric Conversion Chart

VOLUME CONVERSIONS

U.S. Volume Measure	Metric Equivalent
⅛ teaspoon	0.5 milliliter
¼ teaspoon	1 milliliter
½ teaspoon	2 milliliters
1 teaspoon	5 milliliters
½ tablespoon	7 milliliters
1 tablespoon (3 teaspoons)	15 milliliters
2 tablespoons (1 fluid ounce)	30 milliliters
¼ cup (4 tablespoons)	60 milliliters
⅓ cup	90 milliliters
½ cup (4 fluid ounces)	125 milliliters
⅔ cup	160 milliliters
¾ cup (6 fluid ounces)	180 milliliters
1 cup (16 tablespoons)	250 milliliters
1 pint (2 cups)	500 milliliters
1 quart (4 cups)	1 liter (about)

WEIGHT CONVERSIONS

U.S. Weight Measure	Metric Equivalent
½ ounce	15 grams
1 ounce	30 grams
2 ounces	60 grams
3 ounces	85 grams
¼ pound (4 ounces)	115 grams
½ pound (8 ounces)	225 grams
¾ pound (12 ounces)	340 grams
1 pound (16 ounces)	454 grams

OVEN TEMPERATURE CONVERSIONS

Degrees Fahrenheit	Degrees Celsius
200 degrees F	95 degrees C
250 degrees F	120 degrees C
275 degrees F	135 degrees C
300 degrees F	150 degrees C
325 degrees F	160 degrees C
350 degrees F	180 degrees C
375 degrees F	190 degrees C
400 degrees F	205 degrees C
425 degrees F	220 degrees C
450 degrees F	230 degrees C

BAKING PAN SIZES

American	Metric
8 x 1½ inch round baking pan	20 x 4 cm cake tin
9 x 1½ inch round baking pan	23 x 3.5 cm cake tin
11 x 7 x 1½ inch baking pan	28 x 18 x 4 cm baking tin
13 x 9 x 2 inch baking pan	30 x 20 x 5 cm baking tin
2 quart rectangular baking dish	30 x 20 x 3 cm baking tin
15 x 10 x 2 inch baking pan	30 x 25 x 2 cm baking tin (Swiss roll tin)
9 inch pie plate	22 x 4 or 23 x 4 cm pie plate
7 or 8 inch springform pan	18 or 20 cm springform or loose bottom cake tin
9 x 5 x 3 inch loaf pan	23 x 13 x 7 cm or 2 lb narrow loaf or pate tin
1½ quart casserole	1.5 liter casserole
2 quart casserole	2 liter casserole

Index

Note: Page numbers in **bold** indicate recipe category lists.